International Dictionary of Mu Therapy

Therapeutic uses of music can vary greatly from one indiv another, blurring boundaries and understandings across natio lines. This groundbreaking work is the first to bring together international array of contributors into one resource.

The *International Dictionary of Music Therapy* offers mo interventions that range from regional to international, inclu that have never before been published. Essential for both se music therapists and those working closely with the field, it o sive guide to key terms, explained from multiple perspectives to clinical literature. Each entry contains detailed definitic strengthen practice, generate discussion and develop a deep and understanding of music therapy terms used globally. Cove carefully selected terms, this comprehensive reference tool is for defining and exploring the therapeutic value of music.

The ultimate companion to understanding the science and a on an international level, the *International Dictionary of Musi* for music therapists, theorists, educators, researchers and stud

Kevin Kirkland, PhD, MTA, is a music therapy instru University, Canada, and music therapist at the Burnaby Centre and Addiction. He is co-author of *Full Circle: Spiritual Thera*

International Dictionary of Music Therapy

Edited by Kevin Kirkland

Routledge
Taylor & Francis Group
LONDON AND NEW YORK

First published 2013
by Routledge
27 Church Road, Hove, East Sussex BN3 2FA

Simultaneously published in the USA and Canada
by Routledge
711 Third Avenue, New York, NY 10017

Routledge is an imprint of the Taylor and Francis Group, an informa business

British Library Cataloguing in Publication Data
A catalogue record for this book is available from the British Library

Library of Congress Cataloging in Publication Data
International dictionary of music therapy / edited by Kevin Kirkland.
pages cm
Includes bibliographical references.
1. Music therapy–Dictionaries. I. Kirkland, Kevin H., 1963–
ML102.M83157 2013
615.8'515403–dc23
2012050054

ISBN: 978-0-415-80940-5 (hbk)
ISBN: 978-0-415-80941-2 (pbk)
ISBN: 978-0-203-49306-9 (ebk)

Typeset in Times
by FiSH Books, London

My love and thanks to my best friend and life partner, Brent, who also spent many dedicated hours helping to edit this text.

Contents

Contributors

Brian Abrams (USA), PhD, MT-BC, LPC, LCAT, FAMI, has been a music therapist since 1995, with clinical experience involving a wide range of populations. He has published and presented internationally on many topics such as music therapy in cancer care, music psychotherapy and humanistic dimensions of music therapy. His current interests include contributing to the development of the global, interdisciplinary area of health humanities. He also recently helped create a music therapy programme at Trinitas Comprehensive Cancer Center in Elizabeth, NJ.

Anthi Agrotou (Cyprus), PhD, Supervisor EMTR, qualified as a music therapist at the University of Surrey Roehampton, London, received her doctorate from the University of Sheffield, UK, and is a registered supervisor of the European Music Therapy Confederation. Her music therapy publications, emanating from her clinical work, include the documentary *Sounds and Meaning: Group Music Therapy with People with Profound Learning Difficulties and Their Carers*. She is Professor of Music Therapy at the Arte Musical Academy and practises privately in psychodynamic music therapy.

Bill Ahessy (Ireland), MMT, PGD MT, BMus, is an Irish music therapist and researcher who completed his training in Australia at the University of Technology, Sydney. In 2007, he was awarded an MMT (research) from the University of Cádiz, Spain. Bill works in Dublin, Ireland, in the areas of child and adult psychiatry, children with multiple disabilities and visual impairment and older persons. He has published research, has presented papers internationally and has continuing research interests.

David Aldridge (Germany) is a writer. He has published extensively about music therapy, spirituality and health care with Jessica Kingsley Publishers, London. His most recent body of work has concentrated on working with families through his ecosystemic model of distress management with children in distress and suicide prevention. He was a pioneer in writing about research methods appropriate to the field of integrated medicine. His writing focus is on how we make sense of the world.

David Alter (Canada) has over 100 peer-reviewed scholarly publications, many in leading medical journals. He has received over CAN$17,000,000 in peer-reviewed funding as principal and/or co-investigator. He is also a singer-songwriter and has written over 700 songs, some of which have placed as finalists or semi-finalists in international award competitions. He has received radio play in many countries with such songs as *Legend in the world* (Jesse James), *Take me home* and *I'm rolling in it*. He is the Founder and President of Vigour Projects, a not-for-profit organization whose mission is to improve the health of populations through music.

Diane Austin (USA), DA, ACMT, LCAT, is the Director of the Music Psychotherapy Center in New York City, where she offers a two-year postgraduate certificate programme in vocal psychotherapy. She has maintained a private practice in music psychotherapy for over 25 years and is an associate professor in the music therapy department at New York University. She has lectured and taught internationally and her work has been published in numerous journals and books. Diane created the first international distance training program in vocal psychotherapy last year in Vancouver, BC. More recently, she established a similar programme in Seoul, Korea, and her 2010 Jessica Kingsley book, *The Theory and Practice of Vocal Psychotherapy: Songs of the Self.*

Sue Baines (Canada), BMus, Honours BMT, MA in Music Therapy, FAMI, PhD Candidate in Music Therapy, accredited by the Canadian Association for Music Therapy, has practised music therapy with diverse physical, emotional, social and spiritual concerns in many settings. Since 1994, She has served persons in long-term care and persons in crisis with dual-diagnosis intellectual deficit/mental health in Vancouver. Sue teaches piano in the Bachelor of Music Therapy programme at Capilano University.

Felicity Baker (Australia) is an Associate Professor and Australia Research Council Future Fellow (2010–2015), based at the University of Queensland, and National President of the Australian Music Therapy Association Inc. (2011–2014). Her research expertise includes music therapy in neuro-rehabilitation and therapeutic song writing. She has attracted over A$1 million in research funding and received numerous awards include prestigious awards: Australian Leadership Award (2011), Australian Award for University Teaching (2009) and a Foundation Research Excellence Award (2008).

Roey Bar-Even (Israel) is a musician and drummer, who has taken part in different Batukada performing groups in New York City. Graduated at City College of New York with a BFA in music and sonic arts (2001). He is a music and movement therapist, graduating at Lewinsky College (2005). Has worked since graduation at Neve tze'elim, a residential treatment centre for adolescents with psychological problems and post-traumatic stress disorder. Member of 'The

Dreamers', a musical group which creates therapeutic music for children and adults.

Marianne Bargiel (Canada), MA, MTA, has been working for 15 years as a music therapist with children and adults experiencing developmental delay and/or some emotional issues. She earned a baccalaureate in music therapy at the Université du Québec à Montréal (1991) and a Masters in Creative Arts Therapies at Concordia University (2004). She is currently part time faculty in Concordia's Graduate Music Therapy Certificate programme while pursuing a doctorate in psychology at Université du Québec à Trois-Rivières. Her main research interests are psychopathology and emotional perception in music. She is also the director of the Institut québécois de musicothérapie, through which she has supervised a number of music therapy interns since 1996.

Lee Bartel (Canada), PhD, is Professor and Associate Dean-Research at the Faculty of Music, University of Toronto. His current research focuses on music in medicine, including rehabilitation of music perception and enjoyment in cochlear implant users at Sunnybrook Health Centre and research on music and pain at the Wasser Pain Management Centre, Mount Sinai Hospital, Toronto. He is the scientific designer of 25 music and health recordings on the Sonic Aid and Solitudes labels.

Naomi Bell (Canada), BMT, is an accredited music therapist who specializes in work with children and youth on the autism spectrum. She graduated from Capilano College with a degree in music therapy and is currently completing the Master's of Teaching programme at the University of Calgary. Naomi wants to bring her work as a music therapist into the special education classroom, with the goal of teaching non-musical skills such as communication, socialization and self-confidence through music. As a member of the Canadian Association for Music Therapy, Naomi participates as a peer editor for the *Canadian Journal of Music Therapy*.

Lars Ole Bonde (Denmark), PhD, FAMI, MTL, is a clinical supervisor and associate guided imagery and music trainer. He has been Associate Professor in Music Therapy, Aalborg University, since 1995 and is a former head of PhD studies, head of studies and head of department. He is a PhD supervisor and member of the board of the postgraduate training course in music therapy at Aalborg University and Professor in Music and Health at the Norwegian Academy of Music. His research topics include music psychology, music education, music analysis, opera, music therapy in psychiatry, cancer rehabilitation and palliative care. He has written numerous books, chapters and journal articles on these topics.

Bob Bruer (Canada) completed his music therapy studies at Wilfrid Laurier University and was accredited as a music therapist in 1999 by the Canadian

Association for Music Therapy. Bob spent 2004–2005 in St Louis, completing a Masters degree in psychiatric epidemiology. Since 2010, he has worked as an independent clinical decision-support consultant to inpatient psychiatric programmes. He remains musically active, accompanying two community choirs, and is Board President to the Midland (Ontario) Out of the Cold programme.

Sarah Burns (Australia), PhD (University of Newcastle), is a registered music therapist, registered arts therapist and researcher specializing in oncology, stress management and stroke rehabilitation. Her doctoral research investigated the effects and experience of group improvisational music therapy amongst women recently diagnosed with breast cancer. She is currently Visiting Research Fellow at the University of Adelaide and Music Therapy Consultant at the International Centre for Allied Health Research, University of South Australia.

Debbie Carroll (Canada), PhD, LGSMT, MTA, has been Music Therapy Professor at the Université du Québec à Montréal since 1985. An accomplished pianist with extensive clinical experience in special education and child and adolescent psychiatry, she has presented her work national and internationally. Her research interests include the role of melody in developing language in children with Down's syndrome, children's intuitive musical understandings as reflected in their invented musical notations, and the teaching of clinical improvisational techniques.

Michael Cassity (USA), PhD, BC-MT is Professor and Director of Graduate Studies in Music Therapy at Drury University. He is a past President of the Southwestern Region of the American Music Therapy Association (SWAMTA) and a 1998 recipient of SWAMTA's Harmony Award for outstanding research contributions. He is author of *Multimodal Psychiatric Music Therapy for Adults, Adolescents and Children* and numerous articles in journals and books. He was awarded the honorary title of Professor Emeritus by the Board of Regents of Oklahoma Colleges for his contributions as director and founder of music therapy at Southwestern Oklahoma State University from 1981–2001. He presently serves on the Editorial Board of the *Journal of Music Therapy*.

Andrea Cave (Canada) was born and raised in Victoria, British Columbia. From a young age, she showed a love for all things musical. Piano and violin studies have allowed her to play in many orchestras, bands and chamber ensembles. After over two years at Camosun College, she entered the Bachelor of Music Therapy programme at Capilano University, in North Vancouver, BC. At this present time, Andrea is looking forward to her internship and contributing to the field of music therapy.

Donna Chadwick (USA) has been a leader in the field of music therapy for decades. Donna has maintained a passionate devotion to clinical practice throughout her career. An author, international conference speaker, academic programme director, she has contributed over 100 presentations on four continents, has appeared in documentary films and has held national office with the American Association for Music Therapy. A steadfast advocate for music therapy as an evidence-based healing modality, she is as Associate Professor of Music Therapy at Boston's Berklee College of Music. A Board Certified Music Therapist and Licensed Mental Health Counsellor, she specializes in clinical assessment.

Cynthia Colwell (USA) is the Director of Music Therapy at the University of Kansas. Her research interests are Orff music therapy, inclusion in music education, attitudes toward children with disabilities and teacher/therapist training. She currently serves on the Editorial Board of the *Journal of Research in Music Education* and is the Series Editor for the American Music Therapy Association's *Effective Clinical Practice in Music Therapy* Monograph series.

Claudio Cominardi (Italy) is a Certified Music Therapist in Italy, living and working in Brescia. His work mainly revolves around preschool children, researching new forms of musical and analogical languages aimed at intercultural integration, developmental and learning disabilities. A trainer of students and teachers in several institutions, he has presented his studies at international venues. He is a Lecturer in Music Therapy at Università Cattolica del Sacro Cuore di Brescia, Italy and a Member of the World Federation of Music Therapy Clinical Practice Commission.

Liz Coombes (Wales) was born in Cardiff, Wales. She received her undergraduate training at London University and postgraduate training in Wales. She is Programme Leader of the Master of Arts in Music Therapy at the University of Newport, Wales. She specializes in working with children and young people with emotional problems. She is also researching the efficacy of music therapy with populations traumatized as a result of conflict, her initial studies in this having been undertaken in Palestine.

Kalani Das (USA). Kalani's work honours past traditions while expanding the fields of music education, music therapy and professional and personal development. He is a Board Certified Music Therapist, currently providing services in the Los Angeles area. He has also toured nationally and internationally with Yanni, Barry Manilow, Suzanne Cianni, Benise and others. He presents events and training courses. His forthcoming book, *The Way of Music*, examines how improvisation may be developed and used within clinical music therapy.

Jos De Backer (Belgium), PhD, is Professor at the College of Science and Art, Lemmensinstituut campus (KU Leuven) of music therapy and head of the Masters training course in music therapy in Belgium. He is Head of the Music Therapy Department at the Psychiatric University Centre-K.U. Leuven, Kortenberg campus, where he works as a music therapist treating young psychotic patients. He is Past President of the European Music Therapy Confederation. Jos is a board member of the International Doctoral Studies at the University of Aalborg, Denmark. He also maintains a private practice.

Patxi del Campo (Spain), music therapist, fellow of the Association for Music and Imagery and specialist in group dynamics, is the Director of the Postgraduate Course in Music Therapy at the Music, Art and Process Institute in Vitoria-Gasteiz, Spain. He is the author of several publications about music therapy and the director of *Música, Arte y Proceso Journal*. He is one of the co-founders of the European Committee of Music Therapy (1990). In 1993, he was the chairman of the VII World Music Therapy Congress in Vitoria. From 1993 to 1999 he was the Secretary of the World Federation of Music Therapy.

George Duerkson (USA) is professor and former chair of the Department of Music Education and Music Therapy at the University of Kansas. He trained at Kansas and interned in England. He became a Registered Music Therapist in 1976 and was Board Certified (MT-BC) in 1988. His interests include functional music, measurement/evaluation and improvisation techniques. He has served on the editorial board of the *Journal of Music Therapy* and has been editor of *the Journal of Research in Music Education*.

Rebecca Engen (USA), PhD, MT-BC, Neurologic Music Therapist, is an Associate Professor and Director of Music Therapy at Queens University of Charlotte in Charlotte, North Carolina. Her clinical expertise is in adult psychiatry and general medicine. She is a regular presenter at conferences and has published in a variety of journals. Her research interests centre around vocal techniques and habits, with an emphasis on vocal health for music therapists.

Lillian Eyre (USA), PhD, MT-BC, MTA, LPC, is Assistant Professor of Music Therapy at Immaculata University. She has worked extensively in psychiatry and in community mental health, and with adults in private practice. Her research interests include applications of narrative therapy practices to music therapy and clinical improvisation. She serves on the editorial review board of *The Arts in Psychotherapy* and is a member of the Professional Supervision Training Committee for the Canadian Association for Music Therapy.

Gabriel Federico (Argentina), BMT, Medical School, University of El Salvador in Buenos Aires, is a university professor, international lecturer and author of five books on music therapy. He is the Director of CAMINO, the Argentine centre of music therapy and research in neurodevelopmental and obstetrics. Gabriel is Past President of the Argentinean Association of Music Therapy and is Director of Mami Sounds (prenatal music therapy programmes). Since 1992, he has devoted himself to studying music therapy in the fields of obstetrics, neonatology and neurodevelopment.

CharCarol Fisher (USA), MA, MT-BC, holds a Bachelor of Music in saxophone performance, and a Master of Arts degree in music therapy. She serves at-risk families and adults with mental illness in Kansas City, MO. She has developed a unique preventive therapeutic curriculum using hip-hop music. She is an administrator and educator for the Young Jazz Masters of Kansas City, a jazz preparatory programme for inner-city youth.

Susan C. Gardstrom (USA), PhD, MT-BC, is Professor and Coordinator of Music Therapy at the University of Dayton, Ohio, USA. Gardstrom holds degrees in music therapy and community agency counseling. She has worked with adjudicated adolescents, students with physical and developmental disabilities, and adults with addictions. Gardstrom has published in multiple journals, has edited *Qualitative Inquiries in Music Therapy*, and is the author of a textbook titled *Music Therapy Improvisation for Groups: Essential Leadership Competencies.*

Wanda Gascho-White (Canada), MTA, is head of the music therapy department at Zareinu Educational Centre for children with diverse needs ages 0–21, located in Toronto, Ontario. She is actively involved in music therapy advocacy, having served as a past president of the Canadian Association for Music Therapy and is currently a member of the government regulation committee in Ontario. She chairs the Canadian Music Therapy Trust Fund.

Kate Gfeller (USA), Russell and Florence Day Chair of Liberal Arts and Sciences, holds appointments in the School of Music and Department of Communication Sciences and Disorders at the University of Iowa. A member of the Iowa Cochlear Implant Team in Otolaryngology, her primary research interests are musical perception, enjoyment and aural rehabilitation of persons who use cochlear implants and hearing aids. She is co-author of the 2008 text, *An Introduction to Music Therapy Theory and Practice.*

Simon Gilbertson (Norway), Dr rer med, Dip MTh (NR), Dip MT, RMT, is Associate Professor in Music Therapy and Head of Studies of the Integrated Master in Music Therapy and a member of the GAMUT Music Therapy Research Centre at the Grieg Academy, University of Bergen, Norway. He has worked as a clinician, researcher, educator, reviewer and editor in England, Germany, Ireland and Norway. He has particularly focused on relational rehabilitation, neurological illness and trauma, improvisation and the nervous system: central, peripheral and social.

Gabriella Giordanella Perilli (Italy), PhD, FAMI, AMI Primary Trainer, Cognitive Psychotherapist, Dean and Faculty Member of the post-degree School of Psychotherapy and Integrated Music Therapy in Rome. She has been an accredited psychotherapist in Italy for the past 25 years and maintains clinical work in public institutions and private practice. She conducts research in psychology and in music therapy. She has organized numerous conferences and presented scientific papers and is European co-editor of *Voices*.

Stephen Glascoe (Wales) was born in London, England, in 1951 and qualified in medicine in 1974. Achieving membership of the Royal College of General Practitioners in 1978, he has been a partner in an NHS practice in Cardiff, Wales, since 1979. He has always taken a keen interest in the concept of holistic medicine and has embraced alternative forms of medicine, such as acupuncture and homoeopathy. He has been a registered trainer of undergraduates with the University of Wales Medical School since 1983.

Karen Goodman (USA), MS, RMT, LCAT, Professor of Music Therapy, has directed the music therapy programmes at Montclair State University, Montclair, New Jersey, for over two decades while also developing and teaching 31 courses at undergraduate and graduate level. Author of *Music Therapy Groupwork With Special Needs Children: The Evolving Process* (2007) and *Music Therapy Education and Training: From Theory to Practice* (2011). She lectures internationally on topics related to her varied clinical practice and perspectives as an educator.

Susan Hadley (USA), PhD, MT-BC, is Professor of Music Therapy at Slippery Rock University, Pennsylvania, USA. She is editor of *Feminist Perspectives in Music Therapy* (Barcelona, 2006), *Psychodynamic Music Therapy: Case Studies* (Barcelona, 2003) and co-editor (with George Yancy) of *Therapeutic Uses of Rap Music* (Routledge, 2011) and *Narrative Identities: Psychologists Engaged in Self-Construction* (Jessica Kingsley Press, 2005). She has published numerous articles, book chapters and reviews. Her research focuses on feminism, race, disability and psychotherapy.

Hanna Hakomäki (Finland) is a music therapist, psychotherapist, supervisor, piano teacher and PhD student in Finland. Hanna has worked as a music therapist in private practice and as a trainer and supervisor in music therapy education and has over 25 years of experience with individuals with developmental disabilities, children and young people with psychiatric problems and with their families and in special music education.

Deanna Hanson-Abromeit (USA) is an Associate Professor of Music Therapy at the University of Missouri, Kansas City. Her area of clinical and research focus is on preventive music-based interventions with at-risk infants (premature and those living in poverty). She currently serves as Chair of the Continuing Education Committee for the Certification Board for Music Therapists and sits on the American Music Therapy Association Assembly of Delegates and the editorial board for *Music Therapy Perspectives*.

(Ging-Yuek) Robin Hsiung (Canada), MD, MHSc, FRCP(C), is an Assistant Professor in the Division of Neurology at the University of British Columbia, staff neurologist at the UBC Hospital Clinic for Alzheimer Disease and Related Disorders and an investigator in the Brain Research Centre, with a special interest in neurodegenerative diseases and dementia.

Ivana Ilic (Serbia), MSc in music therapy (University Pompeu Fabra, Barcelona, Spain, 2008–2010); BA in Music Education (University of Arts in Nis, Serbia, 2001–2006), works as a music teacher in a primary school in Nis, Serbia, and collaborates with a speech and language therapist in school inclusion programme. She applies music therapy techniques in treatment of speech/language disorders and behavioural disorders in children. She also has significant experience in treating individuals with autism, cerebral palsy and Rett's syndrome.

Jordi A. Jauset (Spain), PhD in Communication, MA in Psychobiology and Cognitive Neuroscience, is a telecommunications engineer and music teacher and a senior lecturer and researcher at the University Ramon Llull (Barcelona). He is a promoter and a writer of the therapeutic effects of sound and music. Their main works published are *Música y Neurociencia: la Musicoterapia* (UOC, 2008); *Sonido, Música y Espiritualidad* (Gaia, 2010); *Terapia de Sonido ¿Ciencia o Dogma?* (Luciérnaga, 2011). In his youth, he received major European musical performance awards.

Cécilia Jourt Pineau (France), MSc, is a French music therapist, certified by the French Music Therapy Federation and the European Music Therapy Confederation. She has a Pediatric Psychiatry Diploma from the Medicine Faculty, Paris V, and a Music Therapy Diploma from the Institute of Psychology, Paris. She does music therapy in oncology at the Hôpital d'Instruction des Armées du Val-de-Grâce, Paris VI, and teaches music therapy at the masters level at the Sorbonne Paris Cité, University Paris Descartes. She completed a hypnosis training for acute and chronic pain in Liege Hospital and Faculty (Belgium).

Shirley Khalil (Canada), MMT MTA, is a graduate of the Master of Music Therapy programme at Wilfrid Laurier University and works as a music therapist in Toronto, Ontario. Her clientele consists of adults and the elderly in long-term care, as well as medically fragile children and adolescents. Aside from music therapy, Shirley is involved in music ministry and is secretary and past missionary for the not-for-profit organization, Canadian Hearts and Hands: A Mission Without Borders.

Jin Hyun Kim (Germany) studied Music Theory at the Seoul National University (Korea) and Musicology and Philosophy at the University of Hamburg (Germany) and accomplished her PhD with a German doctoral thesis on embodiment in interactive music and media performances. She has been Lecturer in Systematic

Musicology at the University of Cologne, Research Associate at the collaborative research centre 'Media and Cultural Communication' at the University of Cologne and at the Cluster of Excellence 'Languages of Emotion' at the Free University of Berlin and Fellow at the Hanse Institute for Advanced Study.

Kevin Kirkland (Canada), PhD, MTA, is an accredited music therapist and instructor of music therapy at Capilano University in North Vancouver, British Columbia. He is the co-author of *Full Circle: Spiritual Therapy for the Elderly*. He also conducts research on music and brain function with persons with Alzheimer's disease in conjunction with the Department of Neurology at the University of British Columbia Hospital. His doctoral research focused on sexual abuse trauma in arts-based research in therapy/education.

Robert Krout (USA), EdD, MT-BC, is Professor and Director of Music Therapy in the Meadows School of the Arts at Southern Methodist University (SMU) in Dallas, where he was named the Meadows Foundation Distinguished Teaching Professor for 2010–2011. Prior to joining SMU in 2004, Robert was Director of Music Therapy at Massey University in Wellington, New Zealand. He has published and presented widely and, in 2005, he received the Research and Publication Award of the American Music Therapy Association.

Colin Andrew Lee (Canada), PhD, is Director of Music Therapy at Wilfrid Laurier University. He also earned a postgraduate diploma in music therapy from the Nordoff-Robbins Music Therapy Centre in London. He has extensive clinical and supervisory experience and has specialized in the areas of HIV/AIDS and palliative care. His research has focused on the musicological potential for music therapy, looking at links between the micro/musical analysis of improvisation and its potential understanding for therapeutic outcome, culminating in his music-centred theory of aesthetic music therapy. His books include *Music at the Edge: The Music Therapy Experiences of a Musician with AIDS*, *The Architecture of Aesthetic Music Therapy* and (Lee and Houde) *Improvising in Styles: A Workbook for Music Therapists*.

Charles Limb (USA), MD, is an Associate Professor at the Johns Hopkins School of Medicine in the Department of Otolaryngology-Head and Neck Surgery and a Faculty Member at the Peabody Institute of Music. He completed undergraduate studies at Harvard University and received his medical degree from Yale University. He completed a surgical residency at Johns Hopkins Hospital. His research interests focus on the study of the neural basis of musical creativity.

Jennifer Lin (Canada), MM, MA, MT-BC, MTA, is Assistant Professor and Director of the Music Therapy Program at Canadian Mennonite University. She holds a Master of Music degree in flute performance from San Francisco

Conservatory of Music and a Master of Arts in Music Therapy from New York University. She is an American Board Certified and a Canadian Accredited music therapist. As one of the Board of Directors of the Canadian Association for Music Therapy, she holds the position of Publications Chair.

Auli Lipponen (Finland), MA (Education), is a music therapist and infant family mentor. She has worked in child custody in Helsinki, Finland, for ten years. Her specialization is in early interaction music therapy, trauma and crisis-based music therapy for children under school age in child custody, as well as family music therapy and mothers' music therapy groups. She is also interested in early interaction assessment, qualitative research and music psychotherapy.

Joanne Loewy (USA), DA, LCAT, MT-BC, is the Director of the Louis Armstrong Center for Music and Medicine. She oversees the Department of Music Therapy which she started at Beth Israel in 1994. She is a Founding Member of the International Association for Music and Medicine and guest lectures at the Albert Einstein College of Medicine and in the Hahnemann Creative Arts Therapy graduate music therapy programme at Drexel University in Philadelphia.

Julie Lytle (USA), BA, is currently a music therapy student at Capilano University (Canada) with an internship (2012–2013) at Beth Israel Medical Center (Manhattan, NY). Originally from Texas, she has a BA in Cultural Anthropology from Wheaton College (IL) and is the 2011–2014 North American student delegate to the World Federation of Music Therapy. She has conducted genogram and ethnographic research while living in Central and South America and the Middle East.

Peter Martens (USA) is an Associate Professor of Music Theory in the School of Music at Texas Tech University (TTU) and is a founding member of the TTU Music Research Laboratory. He holds a BM in Music Education and a BA in Classics from Lawrence University (Appleton, WI) and MA and PhD degrees in the history and theory of music from the University of Chicago.

Orii McDermott (UK), BA, ARCM, MMT, is a music therapist and works for Central and North West London NHS Foundation Trust, UK. She is a PhD fellow based at Mental Health Sciences Unit, University College London. Her mobility fellowship was awarded by the Doctoral Programme in Music Therapy, Aalborg University, Denmark.

Nancy McMaster (Canada), MA, MTA, Fellow of AMI and Assistant Trainer. Nancy is a piano performer, having studied in England in the early 1970s. At that time she also trained in the Nordoff and Robbins method of music therapy in England. Upon her return to Vancouver she practised music therapy with developmentally delayed children. Along with Carolyn Kenny, she co-founded the first music therapy training programme in Canada at Capilano College (now Capilano University) in North Vancouver, in 1976, and has been a core faculty member ever since. Nancy is a regular CAMT conference presenter and performer and is a published author in the field. Nancy has inspired hundreds and hundreds of students of music therapy with her dedication and passion both for the field and for her students.

Malinda McPherson (USA) is currently an undergraduate at Johns Hopkins, where she is a cognitive science major and music minor. She has played classical viola for 12 years and studies with Victoria Chiang at the Peabody Conservatory of Music. She works in the laboratory of Dr Charles Limb at Johns Hopkins Hospital, where she studies motor cortex activation in musicians. She is an outdoor rock-climbing guide and a wilderness first responder.

Beth Merz (USA), MA, MT-BC, holds a Bachelor of Music Education in Music Therapy degree from the University of Kansas and a Master of Arts in Music Therapy degree from the University of Missouri-Kansas City. She is the music therapist at Operation Breakthrough, a family service centre devoted to helping children living in poverty, located in Kansas City, Missouri. Her main research interests are trauma and specifically its effects on self-regulation in early childhood and attachment.

Peter Meyer (USA), BM (MT), MA, has presented at American Music Therapy Association regional and national conferences, the Canadian Association for Music Therapy national conference and Huntington's Disease Society of America's (HDSA) national conference. The latter was published in HDSA's *The Marker*. He co-authored *Guitar Skills for Music Therapists and Music Educators* (Barcelona Publishing). He is a professional guitarist and has taught private and group lessons. He teaches at Augsburg College in Minneapolis and St Mary-of-the-Woods College in Indiana.

Liz Moffitt (Canada), BMus, MA MTA, RCC, is a Fellow of the Association for Music and Imagery and primary trainer of guided imagery and music. She has taught at Capilano University since 1979 in the music therapy programme. She was the first Canadian to become a primary trainer in the Bonny Method of guided imagery and music and currently offers training at all levels. She is also a gestalt therapist and has a private practice with adults combining guided imagery and music with gestalt therapy.

Paul Nolan (USA), MCAT, MT-BC, LPC, is the Director of Music Therapy Programs at Drexel University's Hahnemann Creative Arts in Therapy – Music Therapy Program in Philadelphia and a Licensed Professional Counselor. His 30 plus years as a music therapist include experience in adult inpatient and outpatient psychiatry, gerontology, child and adult medical settings and neonatal intensive care. He has served on numerous editorial boards for music therapy and the creative arts therapies and has served in many capacities for the USA music therapy associations. He is widely published and presents internationally.

Mirdza Paipare (Latvia), MA, is a certified music therapist and supervisor, who currently serves as the President of the Latvian Association of Music Therapy and as the Latvian representative at the European Music Therapy Confederation. Mirdza Paipare is also the Director of the music therapy masters programme at Liepaja University.

Evangelia Papanikolaou (Greece) studied music at the Hellenic Conservatory (Greece), music therapy (MA) and clinical neurosciences and immunology at Roehampton University of Surrey, UK, and guided imagery and music at the Danish Institute for Guided Imagery and Music. She is visiting lecturer at the National Kapodestrian University of Athens and partner of the Department of Developmental Pediatrics at Athens Pediatric Hospital. She is associate trainer of the guided imagery and music method, a member of the editorial board of *Approaches* and founding President of the Hellenic Association of Professional Music Therapists.

Varvara Pasiali (USA), PhD, MT-BC, Neurologic Music Therapy Fellow, is an Assistant Professor of Music Therapy at Queens University of Charlotte, North Carolina. She completed her Master's degree in music therapy at the University of Kansas and her doctorate at Michigan State University. Her research interests include early intervention, prevention, resilience and parent-child attachment/reciprocity. She is a regular presenter at conferences and has published in various journals.

Alice Pehk (Estonia), PhD, is a music therapist, BMGIM-therapist (FAMI), lecturer at Tallinn University, Estonian Academy of Music and Theatre and the University of Tartu Viljandi Culture Academy. Alice maintains a clinical practice in psychodynamic music therapy and creative trainings in personal and organizational development and stress management. She is Head of the Music Therapy Centre in Tallinn. She is author of several scientific and popular publications, including a monograph on music therapy. She is the Estonian representative for the European Music Therapy Confederation. For additional information, see www.muusikateraapiakeskus.ee.

Frank Perry (England) started his musical career in 1964, playing drums in the UK Chicago blues band, the Black Cat Bones, in 1966 featuring Paul Kossoff (FREE). In 1968, he moved to 'free form group improvisation' playing with Derek Bailey, Evan Parker, and Keith Tippett. Frank began his meditative spiritual music in 1968, committing fully in 1974. Published in *Microphone*, *Musics*, *Music and the Psyche*, *Kindred Spirit*, etc. He has given over 300 lecture/workshops produced and 104 albums.

Shay Pridor (Israel), a musician, graduated in a multidisciplinary programme in the Art at Tel Aviv University (2001). She has worked as a manager of social education projects for youth at risk. She is also a music and movement therapist and graduated in 2005 from Lewinsky College. She has Worked since graduation at Neve tze'elim, a residential treatment centre for adolescents with psychological problems and post-traumatic stress disorder. She is a member of 'The Dreamers', a musical group that creates therapeutic music for both children and adults.

Hanne Mette Ridder (Denmark) is Professor and Head of the Doctoral Programme in Music Therapy at Aalborg University, Denmark, head of the music therapy research team at the Aalborg MA training programme and president of the European Music Therapy Confederation. Her research focuses on music therapy in gerontology and dementia care, as well as the integration of qualitative and quantitative research in mixed methods research designs. She is a certified clinical music therapy supervisor.

Robin Rio (USA), MA, MT-BC, is a tenured Associate Professor and Clinic Director at Arizona State University. Before authoring *Connecting Through Music With People With Dementia*, she published articles highlighting her clinical work with homeless adults (*Nordic Journal of Music Therapy*), youth offenders (*Music Therapy Perspectives*) and developing process-oriented therapy practice (*Arts in Psychotherapy*). She has recorded and performs with Synaptic Soul and Daughters of Harriet and is co-founder of Strength-based Improvisation Training for advanced practice therapists.

Catherine Schmidt-Jones (USA) graduated from Rice University in 1985, having completed a Bachelor of Arts in chemistry as well as a Bachelor of Music and Master of Music in French horn performance. She is currently pursuing a PhD in education from the University of Illinois, Urbana-Champaign. She also teaches private instrumental music lessons, develops open-source music education materials oriented for K-12 students and lay musicians and occasionally performs on the French horn or guitar.

Helen Shoemark (Australia), PhD RMT, is Senior Clinician for Neonatology at the Royal Children's Hospital Melbourne and a research officer with the Murdoch Children's Research Institute. She holds adjunct appointments with the Universities of Queensland and Melbourne. Her interests are in developing effective practice for full-term hospitalized infant/child within a family-centred care model. Helen is Associate Editor for the *Australian Journal of Music Therapy*, is published in international texts and journals and is on the review board for the international journal *Music and Medicine*.

Sergey Shushardzhan (Russia), MD, PhD, is President of the National Music Therapy Association (Russia) and President of The European Academy For

Music Therapy. Since 1977, he has been a medical practitioner and researcher, lecturer and vocal tutor. After State Conservatory education, he travelled as a professional opera singer (baritone) of international class and sang with great success in opera houses of different European countries. He has more than 120 scientific publications in the fields of medicine, music therapy and psychology: four monograph, two dissertations, three handbooks, more than 20 discoveries, inventions and developed technologies. Among his achievements are music therapy conception and reflex-resonant theory.

Brynjulf Stige (Norway), PhD, is Professor in Music Therapy at the Grieg Academy, University of Bergen, and Head of Research at GAMUT, Uni Health, Uni Research, Bergen, Norway. He has published extensively on culture-centred music therapy, community music therapy and music therapy theory. He was founding editor of *Nordic Journal of Music Therapy* (1992–2006) and is currently founding co-editor (with Carolyn Kenny and Cheryl Dileo) of *Voices: A World Forum for Music Therapy*.

Lisa Summer (USA), PhD, LMHC, MT-BC, Fellow of the Association for Music and Imagery, directs the music therapy and guided imagery and music programmes at Anna Maria College/Institute for Music and Consciousness in Massachusetts, USA. She was Coordinator of Helen Bonny's GIM Training at the Bonny Foundation for Music-centered Therapies, editor of Bonny's collected works and, most recently, has co-edited with Carolyn Kenny issue 10(3) of *Voices* (2010), commemorating Bonny's life and work.

Susan Summers (Canada), MMT, MTA, is a music therapist in Vancouver, British Columbia, with over 20 years of clinical expertise in long-term and hospice care. She is on faculty in the music therapy department at Capilano University and is the Program Coordinator of Dr Diane Austin's Vancouver Vocal Psychotherapy Institute. Susan's doctoral research through Antioch University's Leadership and Change Program explores singing and voice as a healing change agent.

Melissa Telford (Canada) is currently a fourth-year student at Capilano University in the music therapy programme. Melissa was born in Edmonton, Alberta, and had the unusual experience of being raised all over Western Canada. Melissa enjoys learning about other cultures and has taken her music to many different countries. Melissa's primary instrument is her voice and she plans to further her knowledge of how to incorporate vocal aspects into her music therapy sessions.

Lisa Templeton (USA), PhD, is a licensed clinical psychologist practicing in Boulder, Colorado. Lisa finished her PhD in clinical psychology in 2003 with a focus on mindfulness cognitive-behavioural therapy, the underlying healing and interconnecting aspects of music and therapeutic relationship issues including countertransference. She currently owns the Interpersonal Healing Clinic, teaching mindfulness and educating the community about various therapeutic issues, while also incorporating music into her own life, be it playing, listening or watching others perform.

Esther Thane (Canada), MTA, AVPT, works as an accredited music therapist with special needs children in North Vancouver, British Columbia. Her specialization for the past 15 years has been in the field of autism, targeting early intervention. She holds a long-standing contract with a local school district and maintains a private practice for preschool children to adults with autism spectrum disorders at her studio. Esther has been a music therapy voice instructor at Capilano University's BMT programme since 2003. She has recently completed Diane Austin's first international distance training programme in advanced vocal psychotherapy. Her most recent publication is in the book *Voicework in Music Therapy* (2011). Her chapter focuses on her innovative method of vocal-led relaxation for children with autism spectrum disorders.

Colwyn Trevarthen (Scotland), FRSE, is Professor (Emeritus) of Child Psychology and Psychobiology at the University of Edinburgh. He trained as a biologist, has a PhD in psychobiology from Caltech and began infancy research at the Center for Cognitive Studies at Harvard. He studies brain development, infant communication, child learning and emotional health. With musician Stephen Malloch, he has developed a theory of the 'communicative musicality' of expression in movement and its importance in therapy and education.

Giorgos Tsiris (UK/Greece), MPhil Candidate at Nordoff Robbins, City University, London. He works as a Research Assistant at the Research Department of Nordoff Robbins (UK) and as a Music Therapist at St Christopher's Hospice. He is the founding Editor-in-Chief of the online journal *Approaches: Music Therapy and Special Music Education.*

Jeremie Tucker (Canada), MTA, majored in psychology at Harvard University when B. F. Skinner was conducting his pigeon research and Jerome Bruner held undergrads in awe with his far-reaching insights. Graduating in the first music therapy class at Capilano (1978), she found work immediately in a variety of settings followed by seven years in a veterans hospital. She has led music therapy programmes full time in a multilevel care hospital since 1993. Some of her work is crystallized in her book, *Multidimensional Music Therapy* (2005) and she has supervised over 35 practicum students and interns from Capilano University, Wilfred Laurier University and the University of Windsor.

Monique van Bruggen-Rufi (The Netherlands), MMT, graduated in music therapy in 2006 from the School of Music in Enschede, The Netherlands. In

November 2010, she completed masters studies at Zuyd University in Heerlen. She is a registered neurological music therapist fellow and has been working in Apeldoorn, mainly focusing on music therapy for clients with Huntingdon's Disease. Since 2010, she has lectured on neurological music therapy at the ArtEZ School of Music in Enschede.

Barbara Wheeler (USA), PhD, MT-BC, recently retired as Professor and Director of Music Therapy at the University of Louisville, Kentucky, and was previously on the faculty of Montclair State University in New Jersey, from where she holds the designation of professor emeriti. Her clinical work has been with varied populations. She edited the second edition of *Music Therapy Research* and co-authored *Clinical Training Guide for the Student Music Therapist*. She is Past President of the American Music Therapy Association and Interview Co-Editor for *Voices: A World Forum for Music Therapy*.

Jennifer (Jenny) Wigram (England) studied at Bristol University and the Royal College of Music, London. She is leader of the St Albans Symphony Orchestra and the Amadeus Chamber Orchestra. Solo performances include Bruch's 1st Violin Concerto and Vaughan Williams' *The Lark Ascending*, both in St Albans Abbey, and concertos by Bach, Mozart and Haydn. She performs in the Wigram String Trio, the Amalia Piano Trio and the Cunningham Piano Quintet, teaches violin and viola and whole class string instruments and conducts junior orchestras for whom she often arranges music.

Brenda Woldman (Argentina), BMT, Medical School at the University of El Salvador in Buenos Aires, is a university professor and coordinator of clinical area of CAMINO (Spanish acronym for the Argentine centre of music therapy and research in neurodevelopmental and obstetrics). She also teaches music, specializing in saxophone, and is a specialist in early intervention and early stimulation.

Thomas Wosch (Germany), Prof. Dr, University of Applied Sciences of Wuerzburg and Schweinfurt in Germany, is head of music therapy in BA social work, director of MA developmental and dementia music therapy, research group in music therapy and emotion and in music therapy assessment-tools. He is co-editor of www.voices.no and is a clinician in acute adult psychiatry, with teaching and research projects all over Europe, the USA and Australia. He has authored three books and some 30 articles about several topics of music therapy.

Laurel Young (Canada), PhD, MTA, is an Assistant Professor of Music Therapy in the Creative Arts Therapies Department at Concordia University in Montreal, Canada. She has extensive clinical experience in various areas including geriatrics/dementia, cancer, HIV, palliative care, community mental health and developmental disabilities. She is a certified practitioner of the Bonny Method of

Guided Imagery and Music, conducts research in both quantitative and qualitative paradigms and has published in several peer-reviewed journals. She currently serves on the Board of Directors for both the Canadian Association for Music Therapy and the Canadian Music Therapy Trust Fund.

Ali Zadeh Mohammadi (Iran), PhD, is Associated Professor of Psychology. He received his PhD from Punjab University in India in 2000. His thesis was on the effectiveness of music therapy for persons with schizophrenia. He is the founder of Iranian Association for Music therapy and has published many books and papers on the topic and plays a critical role in introducing this field to Iranian society. He recently developed a new approach called a 'unified model' of music therapy based on traditional Persian music. He is now an academic member of Shahid Beheshti University and devotes much of his time to family therapy and music therapy.

Preface

A pressing but complex challenge for music therapists and those they serve is to illuminate the language and terminology used to describe music therapy as a field of inquiry and practice. The argument that music is ineffable (Portnoy, 1963: 247) does not mean that we must abandon efforts to articulate the benefits of music in clinical and creative therapeutic environments. Victor Hugo (2007: 145) seems to have appreciated the challenges and contradictions of translating art into words when he wrote that music expresses what cannot be said and that which we cannot keep silent. The need to document the wide range of terms associated with music therapy is a compelling frame of reference for the publication of this dictionary. Although the field of music therapy continues to define, explore and clarify its terms, endeavours to integrate the field as a whole are ongoing. Gary Ansdell (1997) calls for the understanding of music in therapy as process rather than structure, in which affect and meaning are intimately, personally and culturally connected; a process that may be individually experienced but is largely participatory and social; where music is performed, improvised and lived, as well as notated and reproduced. Above all, Ansdell (1997) continues, music is deeply and, in many ways, uniquely and exquisitely human.

The idea for a dictionary of music therapy emerged after I was introduced to Routledge's *Dictionary of Art Therapy* (Wood, 2011). As I scanned through its rich variety of terms, I realized the need for a parallel resource for music therapy. I had many wonderings: what working definitions of terms do music therapists routinely use? Do we all have similar points of reference when we talk about matching? What are music therapists' understandings of metaphor? What perspectives and bodies of knowledge inform their conceptual understandings of specific words? When and to what extent are these understandings challenged or uncritically accepted? How do local and personalized phrases and concepts influence everyday practice among music therapists around the globe? What novel and emerging terms speak to developing views of music as therapy?

After reflecting on questions of this type and undertaking further research, I drafted a formal proposal for the *International Dictionary of Music Therapy*. Developing the proposal itself raised many questions: how to develop an initial list of dictionary entries, how to draft comprehensive yet concise definitions for each term and how to identify potential contributors? What credentials, skills, backgrounds and personal experiences should be considered among potential contributors? I formulated a rationale for a music therapy dictionary, drafted an initial list of entries and developed a contact list of specialists in the field.

My proposal for a dictionary of music therapy was accepted by Routledge and the initial call for contributors was sent out. I contacted practitioners and scholars and those whose interests serve as orienting frames of reference for the field. Individuals who had presented or published on music therapy topics and areas of inquiry both traditional and novel were contacted first. I invited suggestions for other contributors and entry topics. The response was one of enthusiasm. Over the next several months, a widening circle of contributors emerged. Many, though not all, had published and/or presented on specific music therapy themes. Others had an invaluable working knowledge of the field gleaned from clinical practice or training. Some offered a broader philosophical understanding of terms. Other contributors had more specific and pragmatic interests and areas of research and scholarship. Some writers offered terms they had coined themselves.

A personal editorial ambition was to move beyond my own understandings and scope of music therapy practice to create a culturally inclusive professional resource. I began to realize, as I received entries from around the world, that some music therapy terms have a relatively common and consistent usage, while other terms have very diverse, sometimes unique, even contradictory understandings. Such variety reflects contrasting geographies, as well as divergent landscapes of personal understanding and interpretation. It confirmed the need to maximize global representation. It also highlighted the need for a text such as this one. I strove to move beyond a solely North American lens of music therapy, seeking out practitioners and scholars in other countries, regions and contexts. I expanded my list of contributors by sending email invitations to faraway places and by reading through numerous additional proceedings, articles, research studies and Internet sites.

Assembling a dictionary of international scope had its curiosities and concerns. One of these was the use of English as a medium of expression and scholarship. Although many contributors were fluent in English, some had very little English. Communication in such instances called for utmost attention to accuracy and understanding, so that nothing would be lost in translation. Definitions had to be reciprocally edited and verified. In the process of generating and reconstructing text, a sense of mindfulness and community began to emerge, which again reiterated the need for a dictionary of this type. Contributions from different world regions offered not only formal definitions of terms common to music therapists in specific countries but also terms that were uniquely local and individual.

Music therapy, nationally and internationally, has become a field rich with interventions both emerging and traditional within varied populations and settings. With a vast number of terms and the need for brevity, keeping each dictionary entry concise yet informative was another challenge. The focus in this dictionary is on terms, models, founders and methods that can typically be applied to a range of client needs. This was done to avoid a prescriptive and pedantic approach to music therapy. A concern here is that the language of one therapeutic method, technique, or intervention itself might become reified and therefore defined as 'only this'. However, certain methods particular to a given population are provided, since a therapeutic approach, style or tool is not a template that fits all clients at all times.

The reader will also encounter entries which, on the surface, may seem to have little to do with music therapy, yet are crucial to its research, practice, and ethics. Some of these terms draw on principles and understandings of inclusive practice and social justice. Entries such as gender, race, and human rights emphasize dignity and respect for all clients and are central to inclusive care.

Readers will also find some entries authored by music therapy students. Perhaps a word is warranted about this, as it is sometimes contentious as to who is considered qualified to be an academic. I believe it is good mentorship to involve music therapy students in the process of academic writing. While I honour and celebrate the voices of well-established music therapists and other professionals who are passionate about music and its salutary effects, I also believe that scholarship is best acquired and cultivated during a student's formal preparation for professional practice; hence, the inclusion of young and emerging authors along with their mentors.

Deciding whether or not to include the names of prominent and influential music therapists as self-standing dictionary entries was a tension I faced in the preparation of this resource. Should I attempt to identify key figures in the field and risk overlooking and excluding others? Was it appropriate to focus primarily on individuals whose life stories and contributions were a testament to the history and development of music therapy? I decided that it was not only desirable but essential to identify and acknowledge those individuals whose lives inspire and bear testament to the ways in which music therapy is understood and embodied today. Their legacies must be remembered, written and celebrated. Sadly, it was often difficult to find biographical information on persons who were and continue to be vital forces in shaping and informing music therapy.

Some research terms have been included in this dictionary because research is a vital part of effective music therapy. There is not an exhaustive listing of these references, as the entire dictionary could be filled with research terminology. Texts such as Barbara Wheeler's (2005) *Music Therapy Research* offer a comprehensive overview of this topic. The reader will also find several regions of the brain defined, along with some evidence cited from the literature on music's role in each area of the brain. This information is by no means fully comprehensive and is ever-changing as new studies are conducted, yet it is vital to have an understanding of the brain's amazing relationship with music. 'It's like the brain is on fire when you're listening to music', said neuroscientist Istvan Molnar-Szakacs (Gaidos, 2010: 25–26). He continues, 'In terms of brain imaging, studies have shown listening to music lights up, or activates, more of the brain than any other stimulus we know' (Gaidos, 2010: 25–26). It seems a terrible oversight not to include emerging knowledge on the intersections of music and the brain.

Each dictionary entry is followed by its contributor's name. In some instances different contributors co-created an entry, while in other cases entries that complemented one another were integrated and multiple authors listed. The majority of entries come with a rich resource of citations that are referenced at the end of the dictionary, should you wish to undertake further research about a given topic. For consistency's sake, 'client' is used to encompass the various terms we use for individuals in therapy, including patient, resident, subject, consumer, subject and participant, among others, with 'person' hopefully being kept in mind above all other terms of a setting or moment. While 'person' may be preferred, 'client' is used for the sake of clarity, to distinguish between the actions of the therapist and the needs of those we serve.

May this resource be a living text that represents a beginning for the collective documentation and sharing of music therapy practice from diverse international perspectives. My hope is that each definition will provide the reader with a starting place that will deepen your understanding, spark your imagination and inform your work and play. I encourage readers to view entries not as blocks of concrete but as stepping stones towards ongoing inquiry, critique, experimentation and imaginative engagement. Music, common to all cultures and said to have existed before or alongside language, has developed into a profession practiced in numerous countries and, with it, a multitude of terms that are essential to understanding the science and the art of music's therapeutic values. I invite you to take a journey into the expansive and expressive world of music therapy.

References

Ansdell, G. (1997) What has the New Musicology to say to music therapy? *British Journal of Music Therapy*, 11: 36–44.

Gaidos, S. (2010) More than a feeling: emotionally evocative, yes, but music goes much deeper. *Science News*, 178(4): 24–29.

Hugo, V. (2007) *Hugo's Works: William Shakespeare*, 19. Rockville, MD: Wildside Press.

Wheeler, B. L. (ed.) (2005) *Music Therapy Research*. Gilsum, NH: Barcelona Publishers.

Wood, C. (ed.) (2011) *Navigating Art Therapy: A therapist's companion*. New York: Routledge.

Acknowledgements

My thanks to Joanne Forshaw of Routledge for her enthusiasm and guidance with the premise and development of this text. My sincere gratitude to all of those who contributed to the content of this dictionary, who took the time to craft definitions that articulate, expand and explore our understanding of music as therapy.

Abbreviations

The following abbreviations are used throughout the book:

AMTA	American Music Therapy Association
APMT	Association of Professional Music Therapists (UK)
BSMT	British Society for Music Therapy
CAMT	Canadian Association for Music Therapy
dB	decibels
GIM	The Bonny Method of Guided Imagery and Music
Hz	Hertz
MT	music therapy
mt	music therapist
mts	music therapists
NAMT	National Association for Music Therapy (now AMTA)
N-R	Nordoff-Robbins
NRMT	Nordoff–Robbins Music Therapy
USA	United States of America
WFMT	World Federation of Music Therapy

List of entries

Entries

a capella

From the Italian, meaning 'in the manner of the chapel', this phrase refers to unaccompanied choral singing. *A capella* may be used by an *mt* when attempting to communicate with a client in an individual session when singing in a lullaby or to create an intimate ambience. *A capella* is also used in vocal psychotherapy and in vocal improvisation (Austin, 2009). Toning, typically done without accompaniment and therefore a form of *a capella*, is an MT centring practice that can be performed individually in a client–therapist dyad or in a group (Keyes, 1973). Participant(s) sing extemporaneously, using various tones that are usually not predetermined. (*Lillian Eyre*)

acknowledgement

A powerful, simple way of reaching clients, including those in institutional settings, acknowledgement involves saying a client's name, making eye contact and offering a short greeting at each and every encounter in and out of sessions. It may take months to develop rapport but acknowledgement is often a key component of this connection. (*Jeremie Tucker*)

acoustic ecology

Sound's capacity to reveal information as a means of understanding the world. What we hear gives insight into cultural, social and technological aspects of place and time. R. Murray Schafer (in Goff, 2012), Canadian composer and educator, proposes an ecological lens to examine the growing problems of noise and its impact on environmental design. Acoustic ecology examines how living things create or affect their aural environment and how, in turn, that environment influences living things. (*Kevin Kirkland*)

acoustic scene analysis

The process of perceptual organization that takes place in the brain to derive meaning out of complex sound environments (Bregman, 1990). This mental representation proceeds with gestalt principles that are at in good part innate and are similar to those found in the visual modality. The global mass of sounds is segregated into acoustic units that share similarity and/or proximity, thus tending to originate from the same location or auditory source. In acoustic scene analysis, auditory streams emerge from the horizontality and verticality of music. For example, sequential grouping generates rhythms and melodic form while simultaneous sounds create the sensory experience of timbre and degree of consonance. This phenomenon is at the base of musical competencies generally observed in non-musicians. Such competencies may include memorizing melodies, anticipating harmonic resolutions or moving coherently to specific metrics. These same perceptual rules that influence acoustic scene analysis also prevail in the processing of psychoacoustic parameters in speech. (*Marianne Bargiel*)

action research

Action research refers to a variety of collaborative research practices with goals ranging from practical problem solving to societal transformation. Action-research projects often entail the use of qualitative research methods but quantitative methods are feasible, depending on situational needs and interests. Action research typically involves team work in 'action–reflection cycles' (Reason and Bradbury, 2006) where various steps of the research process are seen in relation to real-world problems. A specific tradition of action research stressing anti-oppressive processes is called participatory action research (PAR). Central elements in this tradition are: active lay participation in the research process; empowerment of participants; sociocultural change as part of the research agenda; linkage of theory, practice and research; and application of a broad conception of knowledge (Stige, 2005). Processes and results are not evaluated in cognitive terms only but also as emerging and embodied processes of change in context. Action research is highly relevant in MT, both because of the practical and aesthetic basis of the discipline and profession and because of societal challenges such as marginalization facing many clients and participants. (*Brynjulf Stige*)

active group music therapy (AGMT)

Based on the use of musical instruments and/or voice in therapeutic group work. Clients are involved in improvisational, interpretative or compositional activities (Bruscia, 1987b; Wigram, 2004), including free or referential instrumental or voice improvisations, song writing, musical role playing, structured musical activities and musical productions. AGMT can be applied to several functional areas such as social skills, management of emotions, self-awareness, coping skills, gross and fine motor skills, speech/language skills and self-expression, recreation skills, creativity development, teamwork and effective communication improvement. AGMT can be used on all levels of ability or disability and with individuals in all ages (e.g. groups for psychiatric clients; groups for children or adults with developmental, learning or neurological disabilities; groups for elderly people; groups for traumatized refugees; self-development groups; institutional teamwork). Interventions focus on needs and objectives of the particular target group. The most evolved MT methods that include AGMT techniques are analytical MT (Priestley, 1975, 1994) used within the boundaries of music psychotherapy and Nordoff–Robbins' creative MT (Nordoff and Robbins, 2004, 2007) habitually used for children and adolescents with learning disabilities such as autism. (*Alice Pehk*)

active music listening

Listening to music is considered to be an enacted exploration of the world. It embraces spatial and locational orientations of sounds and experiences of temporally patterned sounds as dynamic forms of vitality. Rhythmic, corporeal reactions to music already shown in infants indicate that active music listening is not merely based on an enacted mental process but rather on its embodiment. In infant MT, rhythmically coordinated synchronization between the lullaby sung by the caregiver and the infant's corporeal reactions is conceived of as a phenomenon that emerges through the infant's exploration of interpersonal communication. (*Jin Hyun Kim*)

active music therapy

A client's active musical engagement in the therapeutic process. Often this engagement is improvisation based. The improvisation may be thematic or not and may be played on the client's instrument of choice. The *mt* may accompany the improvisation with therapeutic intention based on the client's needs. The client's engagement with and response to music are symbolic of how that individual handles new situations, challenges, stressors, subconscious conflicts, and interactions. Active MT may be considered the musical version of free association. *(Kevin Kirkland)*

activity therapy

Traditionally used to engage even the most vulnerable clients in activities such as cooking, exercise, craft, artwork and music making (Montgomery, 2002). Activity therapy was introduced as group therapy for children by Slavson and Schiffer (1975) and is particularly useful with latency-aged children in an MT group (Goodman, 2007). Within the context of adult psychotherapy, activity therapy has been linked to a product-oriented group (Wolberg, 1977). (*Karen Goodman*)

adapted instruments

Usually refers to modifications that facilitate accessible music making with non-symphonic instruments for persons who have physical limitations. The modifications are designed by an *mt*, often in collaboration with an occupational or physical therapist, and are uniquely constructed to suit the client's physical capabilities and treatment objectives. Adaptive devices include but are not limited to straps, gloves, stands, positional aids, grips/handles and suspension frames. Clients who benefit from adapted instruments are those who have cerebral palsy, neurologic disorders, missing limbs, brain injury or other motor impairment (Clark and Chadwick, 1980). (*Donna Chadwick*)

adapting lyrics

Familiar songs are often (partly) rewritten to become personalized reflections of clients and/or their families. This technique can be used with all ages of clients. Highly familiar songs with patterned structures are often preferred, as they allow patients to easily and spontaneously create their own verses and, in this process, identify themselves, their dreams, memories and hopes. (*Monique van Bruggen-Rufi*)

advance music directive (AMD)

An advance healthcare planning document completed by a client in consultation with an *mt* while the client is well. Introduced by Chadwick and Wacks (2005), the AMD is the only music-specific healthcare directive. It serves those who consider music essential to their quality of life. As in all advance directives (healthcare proxy, power of attorney, living will), the words in the AMD are the writer's voice in the event that a client is rendered unable to speak or to make decisions at a future time. In the AMD, the writer may choose particular genres, titles and artists of music selections and specify how to use them. Music that relaxes or energizes is often requested. Most likely, a person's AMD will be called into use during a health crisis. The *mt* ensures that the directive is applied accurately and thoughtfully, in keeping with a client's wishes. (*Donna Chadwick*)

aesthetic music therapy (AeMT)

A model that considers clinical focus from a musicological and compositional perspective. It is primarily an improvisational approach that views musical dialogue between client and therapist as the primary evaluation and assessment tool. Interpretation comes from an understanding of musical structures and how they are balanced with the non-musical foci of aims, objectives and outcomes. Integrating the development of clinical musicianship and musical science are essential to AeMT. Elements of this development include: listening; applications of aesthetics, music analysis and musicology; musical form and clinical form; understanding of seminal works; therapeutic relationship and aesthetics (Lee, 2003). Central to AeMT is the idea of analyzing pre-composed music with the aim of extracting components and styles for advancing the range and aesthetic quality of clinical improvisation (Lee and Houde, 2011). AeMT defines all that is musical in MT and advocates that therapists consider the quality of music they bring to their work, whatever their theoretical or clinical backgrounds, with the greatest respect of care. (*Colin Andrew Lee*)

aesthetic sensitivity

Reimer (1970: 82) describes aesthetic sensitivity as the capacity to have aesthetic experiences, to be able to perceive aesthetically and react aesthetically. In MT, this perception and reaction may be a primary function of therapy related to the cultivation of beauty and Nordoff–Robbin's 'music child' concept (Nordoff and Robbins, 2007). Reimer (1970) argues that we need 'to develop the aesthetic sensitivity to music of all people regardless of their individual levels of musical talent, for their own personal benefit, for the benefit of society which needs an active cultural life, for the benefit of the art of music' (p. 112). (*Kevin Kirkland*)

affect

An important concept in psychoanalysis first mentioned in Freud's early writing dated 1892 (Stein, 1991). In the psychoanalytic view, affect has been referred to the expression of the id's drive, whether it is inhibited or not. Lerner (1998) defines affect as being a passive immediate and direct state of pleasure or displeasure that escapes from conscious ego function. In psychiatry, the concept has evolved to an observable response that is the direct expression of an emotion or mood (Andreasen and Black, 1995). Affect is therefore perceived and interpreted by others through the client's facial, vocal or verbal apparatus. In a clinical assessment, the *mt* typically attends to whatever discrepancies, lack of coherences or congruences appear between musical and verbal content and facial/vocal affect. (*Marianne Bargiel*)

affect regulation in music therapy

A skill that develops in the earliest phases of infant life. One view is that, when a caregiver of an infant fails to contain (Winnicott, 1969) and regulate an infant's emotions, especially when rooted in early childhood trauma, one result may be psychopathology or substance abuse (Bradley, 2000; Omaha, 2004; Baker,

Gleadhill, and Dingle, 2007). MT can approach these emotions in a safe, therapeutic relationship. Music improvisation may offer support, expression, reflection and regulation of overwhelming or unconscious emotions through mutual musical communication and sometimes verbal processing. This containing may lead to an ability to regulate the emotions for the client and is vital preparation for work with other possible trauma (Omaha, 2004.) (*Auli Lipponen*)

affordance

Applied to MT, affordance refers to how musical objects, activities, and situations offer a person some possibilities for action. The term affordance was coined in the 1970s by James J. Gibson, who developed an ecological perspective on perception: 'The *affordances* of the environment are what it *offers* the animal, what it *provides* or furnishes, either for good or ill' (Gibson, 1986: 127). Affordances are relative to the environment as well as the individual. An example would be that the surface of water is strong enough to afford walking for some insects but not for larger animals. Affordance, then, refers to a relationship, not an essence. After Gibson, the notion has been used more broadly within several disciplines, including psychology and sociology. In MT, DeNora's (2000) sociological usage of the term has been influential. In discussing meaningful relationships between humans and music, DeNora argues that meaning is not located in the music itself, nor is it simply projected upon the music. There is a complementarity involved; the properties of the musical objects and activities afford certain usages. Meaning evolves out of affordances and appropriations in context. Similarly, the notion of affordance can illuminate how therapeutic change could be understood as transactional process (Stige, 2002b). Musical artefacts, activities and alliances may afford health-related processes activated through situated use. (*Brynjulf Stige*)

agency

In social and cultural theory, the term agency is often used to refer to the capacity of human individuals and groups to act and to promote change. Humans have an inherent, generalized capacity for desiring, forming intentions and acting creatively. Sewell (1992: 20) compares this with our generalized capacity for language: we have an inherent capacity to learn to speak but the specific language(s) we speak depends on the resources available in the social milieu where we grow up. Human agency is thus constituted through internalization and creative use of resources and cultural artefacts in social contexts. Agency is always operating within constraints, then, because action requires access to resources and personal and social capacities that enable use. Constraints are not necessarily constant, however. People do have the possibility of using and producing resources that, to some degree, exceed personal limitations and the hindrances of established social systems (Giddens, 1984). In MT, music can be a resource for agency in a range of different ways, within the most basic interpersonal interactions and within more advanced activities, such as writing songs and performing them with the expressed goal of inducing change in society. (*Brynjulf Stige*)

alternate states of consciousness

This variation of 'altered states of consciousness' originated at a 1973 Smithsonian Institution conference and signalled a departure from the previously used term. According to Zinberg (1977), *altered states* represents a deviation from consciousness while *alternate states* indicates that different states of consciousness can prevail at different times for different reasons and that no one state is considered standard. Alternate states of consciousness are presumed to exist on a continuum ranging from ecstatic experiences of heightened awareness and integration to episodes of loss of identity (Campbell, 1989). Tart (1972) defined an alternate state of consciousness as a qualitative alteration in mental functioning in which the subjective experience of consciousness is radically different from ordinary functioning. The concept of altered states of consciousness became important with the development of Helen Bonny's Guided Imagery and Music (Bonny, 1999a, 1999b). In this MT model, receptive classical music is used in conjunction with imagery and verbal dialogue and their interplay may lead a client to experience an alternate state of consciousness, viewed as a necessity for depth engagement with the Method (Bonny, 1975). (*Lillian Eyre and Ali Zadeh Mohammadi*)

Altshuler, Ira (1893–1968)

Russian born Isaac 'Ira' Maximilian Altshuler, American psychiatrist and pioneer *mt* (Davis, 2003). He received his medical degree from the University of Berne in 1917 and did postgraduate work at Harvard in 1927–28 (New York Times, 1968). Altshuler began one of the first large-scale MT programmes for mentally ill persons in the USA at Detroit's Eloise Hospital in 1938, working there from 1925 to 1963 (Weird Detroit, 2011). His innovative programmes combined psychoanalytic techniques and MT methods specifically designed for use with large groups of clients. He is especially well known for his term, the ISO principle: 'The music is chosen so as to be isomoodic and isotempic, to match so far as possible the mood and 'mental tempo' of the patient' (Farnsworth, 1958: 160). He later trained some of the first American *mts*. Dr Altshuler promoted the practice and profession of MT tirelessly, speaking to numerous audiences over the years and publishing (1943; 1945; 1948; 1952). Altshuler participated in the NAMT organizational meeting held in New York in 1950. An active member for many years, he served on the Research Committee and hosted the 1955 NAMT conference in Detroit. (*Kevin Kirkland*)

Alvin, Juliette (1897–1982)

French cellist and pioneer of MT in Britain, Alvin developed a humanistic approach to MT wherein music is central to communication with the client. 'The

Alvin model regards the music as a 'facilitating tool' rather than an essential agent of change' (Dileo Maranto, 1993: 579). In 1958, Alvin founded the Society for Music Therapy and Remedial Music, now the British Society for Music Therapy. In 1967, she initiated Britain's first MT training programme at London's Guildhall School of Music and Drama (Aigen, 2005a). She is also regarded as an important contributor to the early development of MT in Japan (Haneishi, 2005). Alvin authored several important texts, including *Music for the Handicapped Child* (1965/1978), *Music Therapy* (1966/1975), and *Music for the Autistic Child* (with Warwick, 1978/1991). (*Kevin Kirkland*)

amygdala

An almond-shaped nucleus deep in the medial temporal lobe near the hippocampus. It is an important part of the limbic system of the brain involved in emotional memory and provides input into the hippocampus. Other functions of the amygdala include emotional arousal, fear conditioning and modulating pain response (Bear, Connors and Paradiso, 2007). The amygdala experiences variations when hearing music. Some researchers have found that pleasant music decreases the activation of the amygdala but activates the nucleus accumbens (pleasure centres). When music is unpleasant or dissonant, the amygdala is activated, interpreted as a warning that something is going wrong (Soria-Urios, Duque and García-Morena, 2011). (*Robin Hsiung and Jordi A. Jauset*)

analogical language

Analogy, as the 'perception of like relational patterns across different contexts' (Gentner and Colhoun, 2010: 35), is located in every kind of non-verbal communication. The analogical language is involved in bodily movements, postures and gestures, facial expressions, voice inflections, rhythm and pulse of spoken words, sequences, and any other expression the body is able to do, as well as communication signs invariably present in every context in which an interaction takes place (Watzlawick, Beavin and Jackson, 1967). Since every analogical communication has two linked aspects of contents and relations, their patterns not only should coexist, but must be complementary to each other in every message (ibid.). The central core of the analogy is named as Mapping, that is 'the process of establishing a structural alignment between two represented situations and then projecting inferences' (Gentner and Colhoun, 2010), in order to produce an 'explicit set of correspondences between the sets of representational elements of the two situations, with an emphasis on matching relational predicates' (ibid.). Music, by offering sonic analogues for emotional and psychological processes, provides an ideal means of sharing attitudes and feelings among human beings (Zbikowski, 2008), as well as creative and non-verbal elements of artistic and cultural languages, and space/time structures of cognitive learning. *(Claudio Cominardi)*

analogy

The concepts of analogy, metaphor and narrative are predicated on the belief that meaning in music is constructed; that is, based on context-bound references founded in bodily and emotional experiences that are transformed into words (Wigram, Pedersen and Bonde, 2002a). Analogies between musical and biological form may describe important aspects of 'being in the world' (Aldridge, 1996: 23). Smeijsters (2005b) formulated an indigenous analogy theory for improvisation-based MT. Metaphor works on the micro-level of sentences, images, events and here-and-now-experiences, while analogy works on the macro-level of units, narratives, processes and experiences-as-insight. '[A]n analogy is more direct, is felt as a form of feeling, and does not use an image as metaphor does... When there is analogy, the person expresses their Self in musical form' (Smeijsters, 2005b: 94f). He coined the double conceptualization of 'pathological-musical processes' and 'therapeutic-musical processes', referring to the two core MT analogies. The analogous relationship between musical and psychological processes is found intra- and interpersonally. The analogy between musical elements and existential themes is a core construction in Bruscia's (1987c) *Improvisational Assessment Profiles*. Smeijsters' theory of analogy presents a new and coherent argument for MT. (*Lars Ole Bonde*)

analytical music therapy

An improvisational approach initially developed in the early 1970s by Mary Priestley and colleagues Marjorie Wardle and Peter Wright. Priestley further developed this approach, defining it as 'the analytically-informed symbolic use of improvised music by the *mt* and the client... a creative tool with which to explore the client's inner life so as to provide the way forward for growth and greater self-knowledge' (Priestley, 1994: 3). By creating innovative ways of interpreting unconscious processes as manifested through musical improvisation, Priestley formed a crucial bridge between psychoanalytical theory (based primarily on intra-, inter- and transpersonal concepts of Freud, Jung and Klein) and MT. To remove obstacles hindering the client from realizing their full potential, the therapist works alongside the client to explore the unconscious and allow repressed material to surface, to become aware of and accept parts of the self (positive and negative) that have been hidden, to synthesize energies freed from repressive and defensive mechanisms, to redirect this energy more positively and to find a new balance between various aspects of the self. The dynamics of the therapeutic relationship involve transference, countertransference, resistance and the therapeutic alliance. Specific therapeutic techniques are described in Priestley's writings (Priestley, 1975, 1994). AMT requires advanced academic training over several years (Scheiby, in press). Further information on therapeutic techniques, training, and clinical outcomes is described in the literature (Priestley, 1975, 1994; Mahns, 1998; Eschen, 2002; Auf der Heide, 2012; Cooper, 2012; Jahn-Langenberg, 2003; Scheiby, 2005, in press; Pedersen, 2007). (*Susan Hadley*)

anthroposophy

An esoteric 'spiritual science' founded at the turn of the twentieth century by Rudolf Steiner. Anthroposophy (literally the 'wisdom of the human being', from the Greek *anthropos* = human being and *sophia* = wisdom) is based on a systematic phenomenological study of the spiritual nature of humanity and the cosmos, and therefore focuses on knowledge gained through everyday experience. An influential movement of social, cultural and spiritual renewal, Anthroposophy has a strong impact on many spheres of life, especially on education, medicine, agriculture and the arts. In the 1950s, anthroposophical MT began as an approach where the use of instruments, scales and intervals is based on Steiner's teachings (Intveen, 2007, 2010). Some pioneers of this approach were Karl König and Hans-Heinrich Engel. Anthroposophy also provided a context for the genesis and early development of creative MT (Nordoff and Robbins, 1971, 1977). Steiner's ideas about the creative nature of love and the significance of human experience, and his concept of musical intervals inspired a vision that sustained the creative stance with which Nordoff and Robbins worked and developed creative MT (Robbins and Robbins, 1998; Robbins 2005). (*Giorgos Tsiris*)

anti-oppressive practice, music therapy as an (MTAOP)

A social work term, 'anti-oppressive practice is a heterodox, umbrella term [that] borrows bits and pieces from various theories... Marxist, feminist, anti-imperialism, anti-racist, critical post-modernism, post-structuralism' (Baines, 2011: 13). Anti-oppressive practice 'highlights clients' strengths while being keenly aware of the ways that their experience and life chances have been limited and shaped by larger, inequitable social forces.' (p. 16) Characteristics of anti-oppressive practice include, 'critical consciousness raising, solidarity and balancing the voice of clients with social justice, and linking with social movements and unions' (p. 86). MT roots of anti-oppressive practice are present in the writings of Kenny (1982, 1985, 1992), Boxill (1988), Ruud (1998), Curtis (1990), Baines (1992b) and Baines and Danko (2010), although literature linking MT and anti-oppressive practice is limited. A 2011 article regarding lesbian, gay and transgender issues in MT practice and training cites an article employing anti-oppressive practice to support older lesbian women and gay men, exploring invisibility and isolation for this marginalized population (Ahessy, 2011: 16). MTAOP recognizes that power imbalances in our society affect us all and that this power differential is inextricable in MT service provision. MTAOP addresses the problems and challenges clients present within a sociopolitical context, resourcing us to create a socially just future. (*Sue Baines*)

architectural tonic

A way of conceptualizing and thinking musically in a session through the identification of a single tone that is introduced into a session and that acts as the central tonal focus for a single improvisation, complete session or series of sessions (Lee,

2003). When using songs, the *mt* will include one song or a series of songs, transposing them into the same and allied keys, the final song always returning to the tonic base. The architectural tonic may derive from various sources: 1) the client, through vocalizations/songs and/or tonal inferences from instrumental playing; 2) the therapist, in response to the client's playing and mood; 3) the client–therapist musical dialogue. The architectural tonic can appear at the beginning of a session or at any other time. Once the tonic has been ascertained, all musical ideas will relate back to the fundamental tone, acting as a musical backbone and providing stability and coherence for the musical-therapeutic process (Lee and Houde, 2011). (*Colin Andrew Lee*)

assessment

'A systematic approach to the evaluation, appraisal or observation of a person's strengths and weaknesses in preparation for treatment planning' (Hanser, 1999: 95). It is an information-gathering process about the client. Information analyzed is used to generate goals and objectives, as well as to determine treatment interventions. There are three primary types of assessment: 1) *initial assessment* is performed at the beginning of the therapeutic process to identify client strengths and weaknesses, and to facilitate formulation of treatment goals; 2) *comprehensive assessment* is completed in greater depth either in an effort to determine the feasibility of the MT services (Hanser, 1999: 80), or 'when a client is referred to MT services only (as opposed to MT being one of many services provided by a treatment team)' (Davis, Gfeller and Thaut, 2008: 433); and 3) *ongoing assessment* is performed routinely to evaluate the treatment process. Areas of assessment include, but are not limited to, musical, behavioural, motor, communicative, cognitive, emotional/affective, social, educational and spiritual. (*Jennifer Lin*)

attunement

Defined by Erksine (1998) as a neurophysiological, kinaesthetic and emotional sensing of others, knowing their rhythm, affect and experience. Attunement relates to characteristics of the intensity, timing and shape of behaviour; it occurs largely out of awareness and almost automatically. In the process of attunement, perception of the above amodal or intersensory characteristics occurs between mother and infant during an intersubjectivity exchange, wherein the mother reads the internal feeling state of the child and responds accordingly, sometimes in a different sensory modality. It provides a way for mutual appreciation of the other's mental state (Stern, 1985b). Sharing of internal states is possible by the fact that human beings have common neural mechanisms underlying actions, emotions and sensations. Within these mechanisms, are mirror neurons that allow us to match, simulate and understand other's behaviours, feelings and intentionality with intentional attunement (Gallese, 2006). In MT, the therapist gives attuned responses to the client's verbal and non-verbal expression, maintaining attention and warm sensitivity by using active and receptive MT methods. (*Gabriella Giordanella Perilli*)

audiation

The ability to give meaning to what one hears (Gordon, 2005). Gordon lists five stages of audiation: 1) perception of sound; 2) first attempts to attribute meaning to sound through tonal and rhythmic patterns within a context of tonality and meter; 3) interpretation of what was heard; 4) associations with possibly having heard these patterns and sounds before; and 5) prediction or anticipation of what will be heard next (Shuter-Dyson, 1982). (*Kevin Kirkland*)

baby science-based music therapy

Uses music as a tool to investigate how babies understand and communicate with the surrounding world. Grounded in developmental psychology, neuroscience, brain development and early interaction. Uses baby science investigation, results and equipment for the rehabilitation and treatment of infants and other clients whose capacity to communicate, act and understand may be limited or underdeveloped (Go, 2007). (*Auli Lipponen*)

basal ganglia

A group of nuclei located at the base of the forebrain, which are primarily involved in voluntary motor control (often distinguished from the direct cortical motor control of the pyramidal tract as the 'extrapyramidal' system). The motor structures of the basal ganglia include the caudate, putamen (the caudate nucleus and putamen make up the striatum), globus pallidus (a.k.a. pallidum), substantia nigra and the subthalamic nucleus, while the limbic structure of the basal ganglia include the nucleus accumbens, ventral pallidum, and ventral tegmental area. Other functions of the basal ganglia include procedural learning, emotional control, motivation, as well as cognitive functions such as psychomotor speed and executive function. The basal ganglia are involved in beat perception by gauging temporal intervals (Matell and Meck, 2000), as well as motor control and sequencing (patterned movement) (Janata and Grafton, 2003; Patel, 2008). (*Robin Hsiung and Kevin Kirkland*)

beat

Nordoff and Robbins include a clinical MT description of 'beat' in their book *Therapy in Music for Handicapped Children* (1971). Evolving from their creative MT approach, their 13 categories of response provide five groupings of delineations for this term. These categories help the *mt* to understand the active expression of beat in clinical assessment and treatment. Bruscia (1987c) offers a detailed clinical analysis of beat and rhythm in the appendix of his 'improvisational assessment profiles'. He presents 13 rhythmic scales of assessment, each demarcated by five descriptors. These scales and their descriptors offer the *mt* insight into clinical connotations of beat patterns and styles. (*Sue Baines*)

Benenzon model of music therapy

A primarily psychoanalytic model that seeks to break isolation through the ISO (Identità Sonora) principle, relational treatment, and communication through an intermediary object, usually a musical instrument. The ISO principle affirms the constellation of sounds that are unique to each individual's sense of identity. The Benenzon model was nominated as one of the five most important models of MT at the IX World Congress of Music Therapy held in Washington, USA in November 1999. (*Kevin Kirkland*)

Benenzon, Rolando Omar (b. 1939)

Co-founder of the WFMT. A psychiatrist and musician, Benenzon became interested in MT while combining his two vocations (Dileo Maranto, 1993: 7). Finding positive results in the treatment of several psychiatric illnesses, he founded the School of Music Therapy in the Faculty of Medicine at the Universidad del Salvador in Buenos Aires in 1966. In 1976, he chaired and organized the second World Congress of MT. His concept of ISO is considered the starting point for understanding the complexity processes involved in the perception of sound-musical, vocal and instrumental expression as well as the relationship of clients with musical instruments. He developed the Benenzon model of MT, one of five models accepted at the Washington Congress in 1999 for client treatment (Dinámicas de participación grupal). He is widely published (1971, 1976, 1985a, 1985b, 1988, 1991–92, 2000) and is an honorary member of the WFMT. He continues to influence the development of MT and is highly regarded around the globe. (*Kevin Kirkland*)

Bilan psycho-musical see Verdeau-Paillès psychomusical personality assessment

biochronology see chronobiology

biofeedback

A process that allows an individual to learn how to change physiological activity for the purposes of improving health and performance. Physiological activity, which can include brainwaves, heart function and breathing, is measured using precise instruments which provide 'feedback' or information for the user. This feedback, combined with changes in thinking, emotions and behaviour, can support desired physiological changes. Bio-guided music therapy (BGMT) combines biofeedback and MT to enhance feedback information. The *mt*'s role in BGMT is to create a physical environment, to improvise musically to reflect the client's current state and to recognize, interpret and respond to significant events during the process. For clients with attention deficit hyperactive disorder, reducing theta waves can increase focus and concentration. Clients can learn to control their theta waves through musical tones that are directly related to their theta amplitude. A music therapist will help the client to choose a piece of music that will serve as a musical base, then the theta waves will be assigned tones that compliment the musical base. As theta increases, the audio tones elevate in pitch and as theta decreases, the tones descend in pitch. Clients are encouraged to lower the pitch, gaining immediate feedback and therefore learning to control theta waves. Clients typically train two to three times a week for 35–45 minutes at a time (Miller, 2011). (*Melissa Telford*)

biomedical music therapy

Describes a theoretical model of MT which suggests that music's influence on the brain and other structures of the human body provide the foundation for therapeutic applications within a medical framework (Taylor, 1997). This model is supported by quantitative research and clinical applications. The term was first introduced in 1987 during the NAMT Conference in San Francisco (Taylor, 1997), although early leaders such as Gaston (1968) and Sears (1968) began to connect MT to a medical model in the second half of the twentieth century. To strengthen existing knowledge into the biological applications of music as therapy and to prepare clinicians to use music in medical settings, information about music-induced changes in the body was collated, using physiological parameters such as respiratory rate and blood pressure. The paradigm of biomedical music therapy was well established in the 1990s within the context of brain neuroplasticity, according to which, music interacts with the brain within a reciprocal relationship, therefore inducing changes in brain function by stimulating complex cognitive, affective and sensorimotor processes that can be generalized and transferred to non-musical therapeutic applications (Thaut, 2005). (*Evangelia Papanikolaou*)

blues

A traditional song structure based on the I, IV, and V chords in music. Blues form originated in the late nineteenth century in African-American communities and is prominent in both jazz and rock 'n' roll music. In MT, the blues form is a strong basis for both improvised and composed songs, using a structure that is repetitive, familiar and accessible to most clients. The pattern for four-beat twelve-bar blues goes: I, IV, I, I / I, IV, I, I / V, IV, I, V, then repeats. Altered tones like the flat three and flat five add to the blues mood. The lyrics of a twelve-bar blues song often follow what is known as an AAB pattern. 'A' refers to the first and second four-bar verse and 'B' is the third four-bar verse. In a twelve-bar blues, the first and second lines are repeated and the third line is a response to them – often with a twist, then the fourth line finishes the thought. (*Naomi Bell*)

Bonny, Helen Lindquist (1921–2010)

Educator, researcher and innovator, Helen Bonny was one of the twentieth century's most influential *mts*. She received degrees from Oberlin College Conservatory (1943), the University of Kansas (1968) and the Union Institute and College (1976). She was Director of MT at Catholic University (1975–1979), and she directed two institute trainings: the Institute for Consciousness and Music (1972–1979) and the Bonny Foundation for Music-Centered Therapies (1988–2000). Bonny researched the effects of classical music on imagery at the Maryland Psychiatric Research Center. Her research culminated in her primary innovation, Guided Imagery and Music (GIM) in 1970. GIM, also called the Bonny Method, is a humanistic/transpersonal method of music psychotherapy that uses programmes of evocative classical music for psychological and spiritual transformation (Bonny, 2002). Bonny was a skilled violinist, whose passion for classical music led her to advocate for a music-centred approach in which aesthetic considerations play a primary role in MT treatment. (*Lisa Summer*)

Bonny Method of Guided Imagery and Music *see* Guided Imagery and Music, Bonny Method of (GIM)

boundaries

A boundary defines the edge of professional conduct and typically regulates aspects of MT practice such as time, place, roles and relationships. Consistency of time and place can help the client experience a setting as safe (Darnley-Smith and Patey, 2003). Boundaries of roles and relationships can serve several functions, including protection of the client (Dileo, 2000). In psychotherapy, Gutheil and Brodsky (2008) differentiate between boundary violations and boundary crossings. Boundary violations are defined by their exploitative nature and harmful effects on the client. Boundary crossings involve the therapist stepping out of the usual framework in some way but the action is not harmful and could in some cases advance the therapeutic alliance and the effect of the therapy process. This exemplifies a more general point: definitions of boundaries are relative to historical context and therapeutic contract (Stige and Aarø, 2012). In ecological and participatory practices such as community MT, norms of *regularity* (of time and place) and *exclusivity* (of roles and relationships) are not always feasible or helpful while *reflexivity* (willingness to consider one's position and contribution carefully) and *expressivity* (willingness to communicate and share insights) might gain importance. (*Brynjulf Stige*)

Boxill, Edith Hillman (1916–2005)

Defined her MT philosophy of working with autistic and developmentally disabled clients as a continuum of awareness, a gestalt therapy term. Boxill (1981, 1985, 1988, 1991, 1997a) adapted this concept through three steps of reflection, identification and contact song, which transpose into awakening, heightening and expanding awareness of self, others and the environment. In her final 20 years, she became renowned in international circles through the Music Therapists for Peace movement that she co-created. She also participated in the Special UN Session on Disarmament, the Consortium on Peace Research Education and Development, the National Conference for Peacemaking and Conflict Resolution and the Global Cooperation for a Better World, among other networks. In 1990, Boxill and colleagues organized the first Universal Music Therapists for Peace Day at the UN, a tribute to the UN International Day of Peace. Boxill was honoured as the first recipient of the AMTA Lifetime Achievement Award in 2005. She pursued her work through projects such as Students Against Violence Everywhere (SAVE) and the Peace School Program: Conflict Resolution and Harmonic Relationships Through the Conscious Use of Music (Boxill, 1997b; Vaillancourt, 2011). (*Sue Baines*)

brain stem

That part of the brain which connects the 'higher' or cortical parts of the brain to the spinal cord and is continuous with it. It is made up of the corticospinal tract (motor function), the posterior column (fibres which carry fine touch, vibration sense and proprioception) and the spinothalamic tract (pain, temperature and itch). It is essential in the control of respiration, heart rate and sleep, and is therefore fundamental to the maintenance of human life (Donaghy, 2009). Severe damage or disease in the brain stem is inevitably fatal. Conversely, catastrophic damage to the 'higher brain', where the brain stem remains intact, may result in the condition known as 'permanent vegetative state' (Martin, 1996). Initial responses to music are first processed through the brain stem, making MT interventions potentially highly effective in working with a variety of client populations whose higher brain functions are damaged (Aldridge, 1996). (*Stephen Glascoe and Liz Coombes*)

brainwave entrainment

A specific kind of entrainment that 'drives' neural firing (brainwaves) with periodic sensory events such as rhythmic sound, flashes of light or the pat of a hand. In MT, the entrainment target is usually in the common brainwave states. There are three approaches: 1) naturally occurring musical events (e.g. individual notes within music; finger-picking on a guitar might play 16th notes with the quarter note at MM = 60, resulting in four notes per second or 4 Hz and causing low theta entrainment); 2) binaural beats: two out-of-tune pitches cause a 'beating' effect at a frequency determined by the number of Hz of detunement (440 and 448 will result in tremolo of eight beats per second). When one pitch is played on the left and the other on the right channel on earphones, the auditory processing system sets up internal 'beating' that drives neural activity; and 3) isochronic sound, used primarily with beta and gamma frequencies, can be created from any sustained pitch with an amplitude modulator to essentially turn the sound on and off at a target frequency such as 40 Hz. (*Lee Bartel*)

brainwave states

Synchronous neural 'firing' as a result of excitation in pyramidal cortical cells (commonly called brainwaves) results in measurable electrical activity typically measured with electroencephalography (EEG) or magnetoencephalography (MEG). While brainwave activity naturally and constantly occurs in all frequencies between 0.1 Hz and 100 Hz, researchers use filters to examine the average electropotential power within specific frequency bands. The most common frequency bands are: 1) delta 0.5–4 Hz; 2) theta 4–7 Hz; 3) alpha 7–12 Hz; 4) low beta (also known as SMR or sensory motor response) 12–15 Hz; 5) mid-beta 15–20 Hz; 6) high beta 20–27 Hz; and 7) gamma 27–100 Hz. When the electropotential power in one of these zones rises and becomes dominant, specific states of being are experienced. Delta is associated with sleep; theta with a state of trance, deep meditation or creative insight; alpha with relaxation; low beta with calm focus; mid-beta with active concentration; high beta with anxiety; and gamma is little understood but is thought to be involved in functional brain processes such as consciousness, memory and retrieval, and signal coordination among brain components. Therapeutic purposes can include the development of desired brain states through auditory entrainment. (*Lee Bartel*)

breathing

A potentially crucial therapeutic focus in MT practice. Achieving a regulated breathing pattern through MT may help to manage pain, reduce anxiety and evoke relaxation in clients (Grocke and Wigram 2007a). Breathing imagery scripts with background music, live or recorded, can target pain reduction in children (Grocke and Wigram, 2007a) and promote relaxation in dying clients (Dileo, 2011). Summers (2011) used modified vocal entrainment techniques to match breathing rates for calming and grounding purposes. Relaxation experiences in MT practice most often begin with breathing or breathing inductions. In vocal psychotherapy practice, deep breathing can be a useful tool for reconnecting one's body and emotions (Austin, 2009). Across populations, MT practice targets respiration and breath-development goals through active singing interventions and techniques. To illustrate, Engen (2005) found that therapeutic singing instruction involving deeper respiratory development improved the quality of life in elderly clients suffering from emphysema. (*Esther Thane*)

Bright, Ruth (b. 1929)

Australian MT pioneer, British-born Ruth Bright began her work in psychiatry in 1960. Her clinical practice expanded to include work with children and adults in a variety of settings, including psychiatry, rehabilitation, and grief counselling. For over 50 years, she has shared her groundbreaking work and ideas, authoring 13 books, presenting at conferences around the world and teaching widely. The emphasis in her teaching and presentations is on practical interventions and techniques that support best clinical practices. Ruth has been instrumental in bringing many 'firsts' to the profession. In 1975, together with Denise Grocke, Ruth organized the first Australian MT conference. She served as Founding President of the Australian Music Therapy Association from 1975 to 1978 and as President of the WFMT from 1990 to 1993. Many individuals and organizations have acknowledged her inspiring and tireless devotion to MT. In 2002, the University of Melbourne conferred an honorary Doctor of Music degree upon her. (*Susan Summers*)

Bruscia, Kenneth E. (b. 1942)

American MT educator, researcher, author and publisher, Dr Bruscia founded the first true North American doctoral degree in MT at Temple University in Philadelphia in 2000. Born in Rockford, Illinois, he was the second son of Nicola and Nicolina Barcelona Bruscia. Following the start of an MT career in NYC, Bruscia earned a Masters in psychology. After his PhD in music from New York University, he eventually moved to Philadelphia where he began his notable academic career in MT at Temple (personal communication, 18 January 2012). He is author of over 100 academic papers and books including the groundbreaking *Defining Music Therapy* (Bruscia, 1998b). That same year, he founded Barcelona Publishers, dedicated exclusively to the advancement of MT. Although most noted for his seminal work in qualitative research, he remained notably engaged throughout his career towards understanding, evolving and demonstrating MT's ability to promote health and wellness. Bruscia received the Lindback Teaching Award in 1988, a Lifetime Achievement Award in MT in 1998 and Temple University's Great Teacher Award (Goodheart, 2001). He is currently Professor Emeritus of Music Therapy at Temple University and lives outside San Antonio, Texas, where he continues to manage Barcelona Publishing (personal communication, 19 January 2012). (*Bob Bruer*)

Bunt, Leslie (b. 1952)

British MT pioneer who was awarded the UK's first PhD in MT from City University, London, UK, in 1985, for an outcome-based study involving children with special needs. He originally studied in 1976 with Juliette Alvin at the Guildhall School of Music and Drama, London. He is currently Professor in MT at the University of the West of England, Bristol, where he leads an MA in MT training and bases his research. An internationally well-respected author, practitioner, educator and researcher, Bunt was awarded an MBE for services to MT in 2009. He founded a national MT charity, The MusicSpace Trust (www.musicspace.org) with its first community-based centre opening in Bristol in 1991. Leslie is a Fellow of the Association of Music and Imagery and a Primary Trainer in the Bonny Method of GIM. He also facilitates group work for adults living with cancer at the Penny Brohn Cancer Care Centre and maintains an active musical life currently as Musical Director of the Bristol Phoenix Choir. His publications include *Music Therapy: An Art Beyond Words* (1994) and *The Handbook of Music Therapy* (2002), co-authored with Sarah Hoskyns. Leslie is a Fellow of the Royal Society of Arts. (*Kevin Kirkland*)

burnout

Prevention of burnout in MT is an ethical requirement in many *mt* codes of ethics. Therapist burnout may be caused by exhausting oneself while attempting to satisfy the inner child of the client; expending energy compulsively and giving to 'save' a client; suppressing emotional pain associated with supporting clients in need; working with clients whose pain reflects a therapist's own unprocessed emotions and personal history; experiencing vicarious traumatization from long-term exposure to illness, disease and suffering of clients; and working in isolation, among other stressors. Mary Priestley (Priestley and Eschen, 2002) said, 'You yourself are your most important patient', a reference to the need for self-knowledge, inquiry and care as fundamental to MT practice. (*Kevin Kirkland*)

call and answer

A variation of 'call and response'. In call and answer, an incomplete call, vocally or instrumentally improvised, is answered with the completion of a phrase (Dimoff, 2008). A form of musical dialogue, it may also involve a statement followed by a response. Call and answer stimulates attentive listening between individuals and can be further developed through the addition of other communicative components, such as emotion, questions, humour, dance/movement, conflict and resolution and empathy. (*Kevin Kirkland*)

call and response

A basic yet rich multimodal dialogue form that is clearly manifested in the earliest mother–infant sound interplay, thereby contributing to a child's overall development. As the mother or primary caregiver and infant intuitively adapt to subtle, dynamic changes in each other's sounds and movements, there is a fluid call and response that has been described by others as interactional synchrony (Condon and Ogston, 1967), affect attunement (Stern, 1985a, 1985b), resonance of the minds (Siegel, 2001), dance of wellbeing (Trevarthen and Malloch, 2000) and communicative musicality (Malloch and Trevarthen, 2009). These descriptive terms highlight the inherently musical nature of human communication that *mts* strive to achieve with clients. This communication involves: 1) responding with unconditional, empathic regard to the client's call (musical or non-musical expressions that may be rigid or impulsive, fleeting or excessive); and 2) helping clients to modify their call by making it more communicative. This may mean letting go of control, finding control or, in cases where the client's expression is fleeting or non-existent, discovering a call by facilitating the emergence of a musical self capable of engaging in pleasurable, growth-promoting call and response experiences. (*Debbie Carroll*)

case conceptualization

A theoretical framework used to prepare counselors and therapists for assessing, understanding, and working with clients, thereby facilitating the development of sound treatment plans and interventions. Stevens and Morris (1995) present 14 key elements useful to MT for outlining a case study: 1) background data; 2) presenting concern(s); 3) verbal content; 4) verbal style; 5) non-verbal behaviour; 6) client's affective experience; 7) therapist's experience of the client; 8) client-therapist interaction; 9) test data and supporting materials; 10) diagnosis; 11) inferences and assumptions; 12) short- and long-term treatment goals; 13) intervention(s); and 14) evaluations of outcome(s). (*Kevin Kirkland*)

case study

According to Yin (2003), when a researcher wants to study a phenomenon in a real-life context, case study research may be a preferred methodology. Researchers using case studies draw upon specific questions based on detailed examination of various phenomena (Stake, 1995). In MT literature, clinicians have used case studies as a form of inquiry to analyze and document narrative clinical observations, evaluate treatment processes and develop conclusions (Bruscia, 1991; Hadley, 1998). Various forms of case studies involving a formalized process of data collection have been used by *mts* (Aldridge, 2005). Case study researchers who use qualitative case studies are interested in developing understandings of MT phenomena as well as the subjective experiences of clients during therapy. *Mts* may also use quantitative, case-study methods for single-subject research to identify, collect, and evaluate the effects of MT on specific behaviours. (*Varvara Pasiali*)

cellular acoustics

Certain sound frequencies may activate or suppress cell activity in vitro (Shushardzhan, 1999). A key goal of cellular acoustics is to study patterns of musical-acoustic influences and find cellular operating frequencies to use in MT, medicine and biology. (*Sergey Shushardzhan*)

cellular improvisation

A musical cell or motif can be used as a short musical idea upon which to develop the content of an improvisation. Dimoff (2008) introduces other musical elements, including rhythm, accent, dynamics, transposition, transformation, inversion, retrograde (played backwards), retrograde inversion (played backwards and upside down), emotional content and articulation (what happens between notes) as well as melody to expand upon the notion of a cell and its possibilities for improvisation. (*Kevin Kirkland*)

cerebellum

Latin for 'little brain', the cerebellum is part of the hindbrain at the base of the skull behind the brain stem that relays information between muscles of the body and the cerebral cortex and controls motor movements, coordination, posture and balance (Bear, Connors and Paradiso, 2007). It is mainly responsible for regulation of muscle tone and coordination of movements, especially skilled voluntary fine movements, such as typing or playing the piano, speech production, as well as posture and gait. However, recent evidence suggests that it also contributes to various cognitive processes, especially verbal working memory and some complex cognitive tasks. The cerebellum is also involved in the modulation of emotion, in the learning and recall of skills and in cognitive aspects of skill development. Among other cortical areas, the cerebellum plays a role in the editing and continuity of processes for images and movements (Damasio, 2010). Musical structure processing and temporal organization of cognitive and perceptual processes in music appear also to recruit networks in this area (Levitin, 2006, 2009). The properties of the cerebellum provide an understanding of underlying mechanisms of MT, music imaging and, especially, neurological restoration and rehabilitation, performed through particular techniques with a specific focus on rhythmic-motor functions related to and affected by music (Thaut, 2005). The cerebellum plays a role in timing and synchrony and helps people to track the beat. It is also involved in the emotional side of music, lighting up with likable or familiar music and appears to sense the difference between major and minor chords (Gaidos, 2010). (*Robin Hsiung, Evangelia Papanikolaou and Kevin Kirkland*)

change

A primary goal of assessment, therapy and evaluation is to track evidence of change. Change can have momentum deep from within such as the inner impulse to play described by Aigen (Bower and Shoemark, 2009) or from the 'music child' identified in the Nordoff–Robbins approach (Robbins, 2005: 30). Kraemer (2006) proposes that, while change may be desired, there is also resistance (e.g. shame) and its unconscious rewards (e.g. transference) in the client against changing patterns and that 'effective therapy harnesses developmental strengths and resilience' (p. 240). Duncan, Miller, and Sparks (2000) propose that the client's theory of change should guide the therapist's approaches, techniques and models (p. 44). (*Kevin Kirkland*)

chant circle

Singing and vocalizing in a group setting, using songs of significance for participants. Chants may be based on a theme, need or event. Additionally, the circle may have a spiritual or social focus. Chants are inclusive because of their simplicity; they are simple enough to be learned or created in the moment. Elements of musical harmony and aural tradition inspire community building through support for a common cause. Daughters of Harriet coined the term 'chant circle' after attending many 'drum circles', realizing that their singing group was providing a similar experience; only instead of percussion and rhythm, the focus was on voice, melody, harmony and lyrics (Dunn *et al.*, 2010). Music therapists use simple songs to bring communities together as part of clinical and community-based practices. (*Robin Rio*)

charting

Charting is the process of documenting client care in a medical record. Client records are legal documents. Therefore, there are specific policies and procedures that *mts* must follow when charting. These guidelines may include directives from a health care provider, government organization, music therapy association, and other internal and external agencies. Charting takes places in at least five circumstances: 1) upon referral (whether or not the client commits to MT, there must be a record of contact with the *mt*); 2) upon commencement of therapy; 3) when significant change or evidence of change occurs; 4) periodically, to illustrate that MT is ongoing; and 5) prior to an upcoming care conference or care plan review. (*Kevin Kirkland*)

chronobiology or biochronology

The science of 'live', 'subjective', 'intended' time in organisms (Trevarthen, 1999, 2008, 2009). Plants and animals 'regulate' the life of their bodies in time and space adaptively. Their actions and physiology anticipate changing seasons and changes of the day and they adjust to what happens 'in the moment'. Animals measure movement in rhythmic units: every stroke of swimming, flying or walking is prospectively controlled inside the body and in relation to how the water, air or land may be moved and offer support. They synchronize actions in the sympathetic companionship of play and for cooperative social purposes. Humans balance the masses of a uniquely complex body in harmonious combinations with a polyrhythmic sense, which Charles Sherrington (1906) called the 'proprioceptive' 'felt Me'. From birth, infants make measured patterns of moving that signal self-related purposes with joy, urgency, panic or pain for what is expected with the same rhythms and dynamic emotions as adults, adjusting intentions, interests and feelings to sympathetic responses before 'facts' of shared knowledge are named (Trehub, 1990; Malloch, 1999; Malloch and Trevarthen, 2009). Stories in music or dance and in prosody of language show a foundation for articulate reference (Osborne, 2009). Rhythmic serial ordering of intentions and affective appraisals is necessary for all cognitions, no matter how artificial and abstract their references may become with experience and training. (*Colwyn Trevarthen*)

circle reflections

MT intervention that can be used in group sessions. The intervention gives clients opportunities to express themselves through physical gesture. Variations include the addition of vocalization and the use of materials, such as scarves, rattles, and/or balls. Each client takes a turn leading the group, while other group members mirror what the leader is doing. The purpose of circle reflections is for each client to be seen and heard and for group participants to honour each other through cohesive nonverbal and verbal unity. (*Naomi Bell*)

circle seating

The physical layout of the therapy space, including seating arrangements, is an important element of MT. Circle seating maximizes everyone's ability to see and hear each other on an equal level, setting the tone for group participation. Circle seating differs from theatre and classroom seating. In row seating, an 'expert' at the front of the group disseminates knowledge to 'passive' recipients instead of acknowledging and valuing the contributions of all group members as co-participants. Circle seating also differs from most performance groups, which often have a stage or focal point for music delivery compared to circle seating where the music and/or discussion are for each other and not for an audience. (*Robin Rio*)

client

A recipient of MT care. The term is used by many *mts,* although references to person, patient, participant, resident, subject and outpatient are also common in health care. The term client is often perceived to be neutral or clinical in nature. Such attributions require close scrutiny. It is often said that the client is the client. In other words, therapy should not privilege the therapist's needs above those of the client. Kitchen (2005), referring to psychotherapeutic contexts, said that, 'the greatest expert on the client is the client' (p. 9). Some might argue that a client with psychosis or advanced dementia is no expert. Yet without the binary of therapist-as-expert and client-as-rookie, we may wish to consider clients as experts on their own states of being. Reframing the therapeutic relationship as one of co-expertise introduces an enactive view of persons as dynamic, intelligent beings with overlapping responsibilities and shared commitments to MT, in contrast to metaphors of clients as consumers or system users. (*Kevin Kirkland*)

client-centred therapy

A form of psychotherapy developed by Carl Rogers (1951, 1959, 1961, 1980) by which the client determines the focus and pace of each session. The basic principles of the client-centred therapist are: 1) listening to and understanding matters from the client's viewpoint; 2) ensuring that a client understands what is discussed; and 3) showing the utmost respect and regard for clients. The main goal of the therapeutic process is to help clients actualize their 'real selves'. A key tenet of client-centred therapy is that clients seek change toward personal growth and healing and have the capacity to find those answers. Rogers initially used the term 'non-directive therapy', replaced later with 'client-centred therapy' and finally 'person-centred therapy'. (*Hanna Hakomäki*)

clinical improvisation

Also called clinical music improvisation, one of four MT methods used in assessment, treatment, and evaluation processes within the clinical practice of MT (Bruscia, 1998b). Clinical improvisation involves a client's extemporaneous creation of sounds and music using the voice, musical instruments, body, and other objects that can be manipulated to produce sounds. While the musical elements that comprise clinical improvisations (i.e. rhythmic, tonal, expressive, and formal) are identical to the musical elements of other forms of improvisation (e.g. jazz, Orff-Schulwerk, baroque, etc.), the application of clinical improvisation differs in intent and also may differ in processes, relational dynamics, and musical/aesthetic outcomes. Various models of clinical improvisation have been developed throughout the world (Bruscia, 1987c), such as NRMT (also called Creative Music Therapy) (Nordoff and Robbins, 1977) and Analytical Music Therapy (Priestley, 1975; 1994). Depending on the model, treatment aims, and clinical setting, the method of clinical improvisation may be used in individual, dyadic, or group therapy, and a client may improvise alone or with others (i.e. the *mt*, treatment group members, family members, etc.). Improvisations may be thematic or referential, that is, created in reference to something other than the music itself (e.g. an event or feeling) or nonreferential, that is, created around and deriving meaning from and in relation to the sounds themselves. Models of clinical improvisation have evolved not only in response to idiosyncratic needs of clientele, but fundamentally as a result of differing philosophies about the role of extemporaneously created music in personal and collective transformation. To wit, clinical improvisation may serve as a medium of experience, in which the client benefits from unique, life-enriching aspects of the improvisational experience itself, or as a means to an end, in which improvisation is used as a tool to help the client attain extramusical benefits and outcomes (Aigen, 2005). *(Susan Gardstrom)*

clinical music therapy

Historically understood as the different MT interventions and methods widely used in clinical settings. A complete definition was formulated by Sergey Shushardzhan (1999) according to which clinical MT is considered as the field of clinical practice that uses MT methods and technologies for cure, correction or treatment of various psychological and somatic disorders, pathological syndromes for rehabilitation and diseases or disorders. (*Sergey Shushardzhan*)

clinical setting in music therapy

Comprises all of the factors that facilitate the therapeutic process, including, the development of a relationship of trust between the therapist and the client and the creative unravelling of the client's inner world. The clinical setting includes: 1) the physical space: appropriate MT room (quiet, of appropriate size, comfortable, containing musical instruments of good quality, which can be easily played by anyone and offering a wide variety of rhythmical and melodic sounds); 2) reliability regarding the physical space: sessions take place on the same day and hour of the week and every session has the same duration. The instruments are laid in the same position for every session (a position which facilitates the special needs of every client) and when changes occur in the room, the therapist prepares the client appropriately; 3) the therapist's stance provides consistency, reliability and stability and includes: confidentiality; focused attention; the non-critical acceptance of the client's condition; refraining from intervention and from giving educational directions; availability to serve the client's psychological needs and not the therapist's; and breaks are prepared for and addressed appropriately (Bunt and Hoskyns, 2002). (*Anthi Agrotou*)

closure

Assists clients with experiences of beginning and end, hello and goodbye, life and death, and relating and separating. Closure is part of the ritual that serves as an important component to group and individual sessions or the end of working with a client. A closing song and accompanied action (e.g. blowing out a candle, waving good-bye) provides familiarity from week to week and is an anchor in time. Closure can heighten awareness of feelings around endings, including previous closure attempts or successes. A group-composed ritual or pre-composed song created for closure infuses significance around closure through ritualizing it. (*Kevin Kirkland*)

Cochrane Collaboration

An Oxford-based international organization dedicated to the highly structured and unbiased review of clinical research across all major areas of health care, including MT. Built on basic meta-analysis methodology, defining features of every Cochrane investigation include an initial systematic listing of where researchers will be searching for trials (e.g. PubMed, PsychINFO®) and pre-specified research criteria required for inclusion (e.g. randomization of subjects, blinding of assessors). By 1995, the Cochrane's ongoing efforts towards relevancy led to the inclusion of patient perspectives, as well as a plain language summary succinctly encapsulating the clinical implications of each review. More recently, the Cochrane has introduced changes that include non-randomized observational studies. MT researchers, such as Gold, Wigram, and Elefant (2006) used the CC to elevate MT's profile. Using Cochrane's features, like the opportunity to publish needed research standards (i.e. protocols) before conducting clinical trials and open-sourced meta-analysis software, MT researchers have better defined and defended the professional boundaries of effective MT treatments (Gold *et al.*, 2005; Gold, Wigram and Elefant, 2006; Bruer, Spitznagel and Cloninger, 2007). (*Bob Bruer*)

communicative musicality

Over the last few decades, the relevance of musicality for interpersonal communication has been discussed in the context of neonate and infant MT. Prelinguistic communication in early infant–caregiver interaction not only consists of turn-taking but also synchronization to multimodal activities of temporally patterned movements that are conceived of as inherently musical characteristics (Malloch and Trevarthen, 2009). According to this research, infants develop in coordinated engagement with musical qualities of sounds and corporeal and facial movements reflect their ability to communicate with others, a phenomenon that is referred to as 'communicative musicality'. (*Jin Hyun Kim*)

communicative vocalization

Use of voice, including vocables, speech, and other skills, for communication purposes. The 'communicative function of speech includes mutual interchange, involvement, and interaction' (Kannengieser, 2009: 5) The word combination 'communicative vocalization' was used in T. Wigram's 2008 presentation materials for guest lectures at Liepāja University. Development of communicative vocalization was mentioned in relation to therapeutic outcomes in the communication domain. Vocalization begins with voice expressions at an early age (Decker-Voigt, Weymann and Bern, 2009). The concept of vocalization, therefore, has close contextual links to the preverbal stage of development in childhood. Since vocalization or voice expressions are discussed in relation to children with autism and developmental disorders of speech, use of voice is essential for the development of verbal communication. (*Mirdza Paipare*)

community

Traditionally, community has been conceived of as a social group whose members live in a specific locality and share values and practices. As societies change, possibilities for community change too. Contemporary virtual communities on the Internet, for example, may or may not represent a shared locality and usually have very few direct and directly responsible relationships that characterized traditional communities. Even if we restrict the notion of community to groups that interact directly, contemporary communities often differ considerably from traditional locality-based communities. In an exploration of musical community, Gary Ansdell (2010a) argues that *community of practice* is a significant model of community for contemporary MT. Community of practice is a concept developed by the social learning theorist Etienne Wenger (1998) and refers to the experience of people engaged in doing and learning something together when there is more than a transitory encounter but less than a formal social structure. More generally, social theory suggests that communities can operate not only as social support systems and vehicles for human agency but, also as oppressive structures. Nevertheless, communities are often considered vital to human welfare and wellbeing. (*Brynjulf Stige*)

community music therapy (CoMT)

A broad international movement and perspective that emphasizes human connectedness, wellbeing and social change in and through music. The roots of CoMT are varied and go back to the emergence of MT as a modern discipline and profession in the 1950s and 1960s. As an international academic discourse, CoMT is a relatively recent development. The first book on CoMT was edited by Pavlicevic and Ansdell (2004). Seven qualities that typically characterize contemporary CoMT can be communicated through the acronym PREPARE: participatory, resource-oriented, ecological, performative, activist, reflective, and ethics-driven (Stige and Aarø, 2012). CoMT exemplifies how human needs can be fruitfully examined in light of human rights, such as the right to citizen participation and the rights to health, education and culture. To define human needs in terms of human rights contributes to the development of a relational and contextual foundation for CoMT: practice evolves in the intersection of human rights challenges and social-musical possibilities. (*Brynjulf Stige*)

complementary and alternative medicine

Group of treatment and/or prevention options that complement traditional medical approaches to health care. The Cochrane Collaboration defines complementary as a contribution 'to a common whole by satisfying a demand not met by orthodox medicine or by diversifying the conceptual frameworks of medicine' (Ernst and Randl, 1998). It is important that MT reposition itself outside the realm of adjunctive or complementary therapy in some clinical settings and interventions with certain clients and be viewed as the primary mode of therapy when it is among the most effective (Zwerling, 1989). (*Kevin Kirkland*)

conducting

Conducting is the act of leading or directing a group of musicians in a performance or rehearsal (Randel, 2003). The one leading, the conductor, shows the beat of the music to keep the players or singers together. Additionally, gestures and facial expressions convey changes in the way the music is to be performed. Conducting is one of the professional competencies of the AMTA (2009). In a clinical setting, clients may conduct as a leadership opportunity or as a re-creative experience (see Bruscia, 1998b: 117–19), in which a musical model is reproduced or interpreted in a live musical performance with or without an audience. (*Rebecca Engen*)

constructivism

Constructivist models of learning emphasize how individuals construct knowledge by interacting with their environment. Each person's unique experiences and mental representations, both as an individual or a member of a group, play pivotal roles in interpreting physical reality as well as moral and social understanding (Taetle and Cutietta, 2002). Researchers whose thinking is influenced by constructivist models of learning often use qualitative methodologies. A primary goal of qualitative inquiry is to understand and interpret the complex responses that clients exhibit during MT. Constructivist researchers seek to understand the contextual meaning co-created by a client and a therapist during MT experiences. Terms related to learning theory were contextualized in MT education and training (Goodman, 2011). (*Varvara Pasiali*)

contact song

Edith Boxill (1991) stated that the contact song – often the crux of an MT session – provides a secure base for the client. A statement of trust, the contact song is about being, becoming and of going beyond. The contact song is typically performed at the start of a session to say hello, to provide context, to set a tone and to bring people together through sound. The music may be pre-composed, co-created, adapted or composed for the client. It typically contains words but may be instrumental. It is often a personally meaningful song of an individual client or group, but may grow to become a significant point of contact through its ritualized use as a primary means of rapport and cohesion. (*Kevin Kirkland*)

contingent singing

The intentional use of singing as a medium for therapeutic interplay between an adult and infant to create interpersonal mutual engagement (Shoemark and

Grocke, 2010). It contrasts with other forms of singing to infants that promote homeostasis or sleep. Patterned and predictable musical interaction which emulates naturally occurring patterns of successful interaction are consciously constructed by the adult singer based on the infant's cues and the intention of singing in the therapeutic interplay. In family-centred work, contingent singing may sustain the intersubjective potential of the infant and carer and provide parents with a focal point for interplay with medically fragile newborn infants. The process of contingent singing in MT is informed by theories and understandings of trauma and interpersonal transaction, including the Dyadic Expansion of Consciousness Hypothesis (Tronick, 1998) and psychoanalytic psychology (Beebe and Lachmann, 1994), which help to explain how the organization of self-consciousness and the development of relational selves are mutually intertwined. (Beebe and Lachmann, 1994). (*Helen Shoemark*)

containment

Term coined and developed by psychoanalyst Wilfred Bion (1978/1994; Cartwright, 2010). Aspects of music, such as structure, rhythm, beginning and ending, predictability, tonality and order out of chaos, are elements that can serve as a container for the client. A container allows room to explore an image, mood, musical dialogue, or affect, while providing a safer zone of expression through thoughtfully applied parameters. It is important to distinguish this method from therapeutic containment of a 'time-out' nature, including physical containment. In MT, music, like a container, can hold a client through a framework by drawing on elements, such as matching, warmth and empathy. Musical instruments and active playing provide here-and-now tactile and audible resonance that is anchored by the therapist. (*Kevin Kirkland*)

continuum of music response

A term coined by Goodman (2007) to offer a system for understanding and anticipating different levels of musical response in a group, from lowest to highest functioning levels. The therapist adapts materials as necessary, using carefully chosen methods for clients in an MT group. (*Karen Goodman*)

countertransference

A jointly created phenomenon between the therapist and the client. Through transference, the client unconsciously projects unresolved feelings and behaviours toward the therapist, seeking the therapist to play a role similar to the client's inner world. Imagine the client has never functioned well independently and projects onto the *mt* the need for an authority figure parent who will tell them what to do. The *mt* has their own needs to be in control and to be a helper, and enters into countertransference, hindering the client from making the steps to independence they need. It is vital that therapists analyze their responses to clients, whether positive or negative, bearing in mind therapists are capable of both conscious and unconscious transference and countertransference. An example Shebib (2011) gives is running over the scheduled appointment time with certain clients and wishing others would not arrive. Clinicians such as Austin (2008), Racker (in Hunt and Issacharoff, 1977), and Heimann (1950), says that embracing countertransference can help the therapist better understand the client and, in situations where it is appropriate to reveal countertransference responses to the client, can aid the client in understanding their effect on others. It is healthy, productive, and arguably essential for the therapist to explore through reflexive practice, peer support, supervision, and/or through their own therapy, countertransference reactions that hold either a positive or a negative charge, because in either case, our objectivity may be limited (McKinney and Thomas, 2010). *(Kevin Kirkland)*

creation axis

An expressive therapies concept developed by Avi Goren-Bar (1997) that follows six stages: contact, organization, improvisation, central theme, elaboration, and preservation. It offers a way of examining the process of artistic creativity in therapy and tracks client behaviours, reactions, activities and attitudes. Goren-Bar lists four capabilities of the therapist: 1) to obtain client clinical information; 2) to reconstruct, follow and report on the therapeutic process; 3) to understand the therapeutic meaning of the process in its various stages; and 4) to find and develop intervention options during the process. *(Kevin Kirkland)*

creative arts therapies

Arts modalities used as intentional interventions 'in therapeutic, rehabilitative, community, or educational settings to foster health, communication, and expression' while promoting integration, self-awareness, and change (Micozzi, 2006: 334). Music has long been considered one of the creative arts therapies, typically including art and dance, and by extension any other creative modality such as psychodrama, poetry, and narrative. Also called expressive arts therapies, it also falls under the domain of arts-based research and inquiry. Medical humanities is a related term that unites the humanities, social sciences, and the arts in medical education and practice (Lazarus and Roslyn, 2003). Willis, Smith and Collins (2000) assert that the arts in therapy have six values: 1) it creates a virtual reality; 2) introduces the presence of ambiguity; 3) uses expressive language; 4) promotes empathy; 5) has a personal signature; 6) has the presence of aesthetic form. *(Kevin Kirkland)*

creative music therapy

Also known also as Nordoff–Robbins MT (NRMT), it is an improvisational, music-centred approach to MT (Aigen, 2005b; Bruscia, 1987b) developed by pioneers Paul Nordoff and Clive Robbins from the 1950s to 1970s. Central to this approach is the concept of the 'music child' (Nordoff and Robbins, 2007), which is used to highlight the individualized musicality inborn in every child who 'responds to musical experience, finds it meaningful and engaging, remembers music and enjoys some form of musical experience, communication, and sharing'. This concept refers to 'the universality of human musical experience [...] and to the uniquely personal significance of each child's musical responsiveness' (Nordoff and Robbins, 2007: 3). The theoretical foundations and practical applications of the approach, influenced by Nordoff and Robbins' clinical practice, research and teaching, are conveyed in their book, *Creative Music Therapy* (1977/2007). Originally developed for children with special needs (Nordoff and Robbins, 1971, 1975), the approach rapidly spread to a wide range of adult populations and settings and today is recognized and practised worldwide. (*Giorgos Tsiris*)

creative team training

A form of group development used in health care settings. Elements of expressive and receptive MT techniques are used in creative team training. Musical and creative activities offer several benefits. They enhance motivation which, in turn, improves the overall effectiveness of the training. Musical and creative activities also produce energy and synergy; develop communication abilities, such as listening and reflecting skills; train concentration and attentiveness; enhance self-awareness and self-observing abilities; increase *esprit de corps*; develop creativity and spontaneity and encourage the expression of ideas; illuminate the avoidance of common patterns in thinking and behaviour and may shift a person's thinking about a health care team, department, or organization and the individual's part in it; allow awareness of stress sources and give opportunities for releasing stress and preventing burnout; and support the development of self-confidence in expression and performance (Hallam and MacDonald, 2008; Pavlicevic, 2003). The group form of the Bonny Method of Guided Imagery and Music (Summer, 2002) can be effectively used in smaller teams or working groups, allowing a unique collaborative experience by playing through problematic situations for the team in group imageries. The Bonny Method also works as diagnostic tool for a team. Valuable knowledge gained from experience may be integrated into the team's everyday work. (*Alice Pehk*)

creativity

To conceive of or to construct something novel or to modify an existing idea, concept or artefact in a new and unexpected way. Although studies about the neurobiological mechanisms underlying creativity are relatively few and have demonstrated varied results, it is accepted that the prefrontal cortex is integral in the creative process. Creativity involves cognitive flexibility and breaking out of conventional patterns of thinking. However, research has not firmly established whether there are separate pathways involved in creative versus non-creative thinking (Dietrich, 2010). Musical improvisation, a form of spontaneous creativity, has been linked to deactivation of the lateral prefrontal region thought to be involved in concentration and self-monitoring, so the deactivation of these areas may allow unexpected insights to emerge (Limb, 2008). (*Charles Limb and Malinda McPherson*)

creativity within improvisation

Creativity appears in improvisation when we facilitate spaces of chaos and contradiction where interchanges of sensation and perception occur, making new communication possible. This leads us from the known as reassuring space full of seductive possibilities (Fiorini, 2010) to the real impulses of doubt and uncertainty capable of organizing themselves into creative chaos. Within musical improvisation, we find a continuous flow of forces that virtually trace an infinity of possibilities and bridges lasting for a moment. A musical improvisation or creation is created by clients: it is theirs, but at the same time it reveals truths related to their surrounding life world. Seeing improvisation as a creative field where a multidimensional network of forces and energies is traced, where the client builds, destroys, moves among contradictions, makes it possible to convert improvisation not only into a product but also into a process where sound envelopment is recreated and multiplies itself into new realities in constant change. (del Campo, 2002) (*Patxi del Campo*)

credentials

A rank or title conferred by a body awarding credentials denoting professional competence to practice MT. While there is a WFMT, no globally uniform MT credential exists. Credentials differ by country and the standards of their respective national organizations. Additional credentials may be required at state, province or other local levels to practice MT, depending on governmental legislation. Credentialed *mts* demonstrate multiple music skills and clinical competencies, have earned a degree from an accredited university and, in some countries, successfully have completed an examination or certification process. The holder of an MT credential is afforded the privilege of professionally identifying as an *mt* by using the formal designated title and letters following their name. For instance, in the USA MT-BC designates Board Certified, RMT (Registered), and CMT (Certified), with the latter two terms valid until 2020. MTA designates Accredited in Canada, and RMT designates Registered in Australia. Postgraduate training in clinical specialties are regulated by their own credentialing organizations. Examples include FAMI (Fellow of the Association of Music and Imagery), NRMT (Nordoff–Robbins MT) and AMT (Analytical MT). (*Donna Chadwick*)

critical theory

The term critical theory is sometimes used broadly to denote a range of nonconformist and/or emancipatory perspectives in the social sciences and the humanities. The capitalized form Critical Theory is often used to denote the approach to social thought developed by the Frankfurt School it the late 1920s. Pioneers of the Frankfurt School included the music sociologist Theodor W. Adorno. Jürgen Habermas and Axel Honneth are the most important contemporary figures of the school. Critical Theory can be seen as a revision and criticism of Marxism, with important influences from humanist thinking and psychoanalysis. Critical theorists emphasize the interplay between social conditions and individual agency. The advocates of critical theory suggest that research and theory should go beyond being descriptive and explanatory and should also be normative, practical and self-reflexive. Other important traditions of critical thinking include feminist theory, postcolonial perspectives, gender studies and disability studies. In these traditions, knowledge is considered to be linked to power and social and material conditions. It is consequently advocated that, as academics and practitioners, we need to take an active political stand. Consequently, emancipation and empowerment of marginalized individuals and groups could be considered a main objective also of MT (Stige and Aarø, 2012). (*Brynjulf Stige*)

crossing the midline

Behaviour that results in reaching, stepping or gazing across the body's midline. Midline movements facilitate bilateral integration for hearing, seeing and eye–hand coordination, important for body-scheme development and bilateral coordination (Ayres, 1961). Midline-crossing integration, or cross-lateral integration, is a developmental milestone typically achieved by eight or nine years of age (Cermak, Quintero and Cohen, 1980). MT can address physical coordination goals through rhythmic movement interventions that develop midline orientation, spatial perception and upper-lower body coordination in children with autism (Berger, 2002). Midline orientation can be addressed through an array of musical instruments and interventions in treatment, such as playing the xylophone from left to right, using one hand or striking strategically positioned instruments. Further application of midline opportunities in MT may target ageing clients as well. Lombardi, Surburg and Koceja (2000: M293) found that 'the effects of midline crossing inhibition on the lower extremities reemerge in individuals 65 and older'. (*Esther Thane*)

culture-centred music therapy

Culture is integral to human interaction. Culture-centred music therapy is a tradition exploring the implications of this statement for practice, theory, and research.

Culture-centred music therapy is in many ways person-centred; participants' biopsychosocial needs are explored in relational and contextual terms. More than as a stimulus influencing human behaviour, culture is understood as a resource for action. This combination of perspectives highlights the interaction between our internal worlds and the external world and between individual and community. Human interdependence is not understood as a challenge to autonomy, then, but as a basis for it. Consequently, how music therapy affords sociocultural participation in and through music is central (Stige, 2002). Bruscia compared culture-centred music therapy to other 'forces of thought' in the discipline and proposed that: 'This will be the force that reminds us that all interactions, musical and nonmusical, clinical and nonclinical, are situated within many larger, frequently overlooked frames of perception and communication.' Related perspectives were pioneered by theorists such as Kenny (1985, 1989) and Ruud (1998) and have become more prominent after 2000, partly in tandem with the emergence of international discourses on community MT, feminist MT, and resource-oriented MT. *(Brynjulf Stige)*

cymatics

A term coined by Dr Hans Jenny, a Swiss anthroposophist who was interested in the phenomenon of cycles or periodicity (with the Greek word for wave being *kyma*) who worked in the 1960s. Ostensibly, a further development of the Chladni plate, it used a piezoelectric crystal oscillator to control precise frequencies to resonate the plate rather than the violin bow of Chladni. Different substances were then laid on to the plate(s) with the resulting vibrations producing replicable patterns. Photographs and films were made of his findings and published. One aspect of this phenomenon was to make sound visible. Dr Peter Guy Manners (UK) developed the Cymatics Applicator. The 1980s version resembled a hairdryer but had a moving wooden rod at its centre. It was discovered that five frequencies worked best through the central rod and these were selected from a computer and played through this Applicator according to tables giving the combinations for each bodily organ. The Applicator would then be placed upon the actual part of the body intended for healing. The basic idea involves retuning the organ to its proper frequency via the Applicator and the vibrations transmitted through it on to the body. (*Frank Perry*)

dance/movement

Dance is an art form generally referring to expressive bodily movement, usually to rhythmic music. Dance, like music, may also be regarded as a form of nonverbal communication. It can be participatory, social or performed for an audience. It can also be ceremonial, competitive or erotic (Panksepp and Bernatzky, 2002). Because music is often time ordered, it is an ideal stimulus for coordinating movement. Knowledge of body parts and concepts of direction can be acquired through dance and musical movement games (Peters, 1987; Michel, 1976; Alvin, 1965/1978). Movement to music also aids basic socialization skills, including peer recognition, team work, sharing, waiting one's turn and the ability to work independently (Kay, 1981). Dance/movement can give clients improved confidence, grace and security in independent movement (Tanner and O'Bright, 1980) and can help to increase sensory awareness, the ability to follow directions, to relate nonverbally and to learn cooperation skills (Wolfgram, 1978). Movement to music can help to improve motor coordination skills including: 1) performing motor movements to a steady or rhythmic beat; 2) performing non-locomotive movements (bending, swaying, rocking) to the beat; 3) performing actions described by song lyrics; 4) learning and performing dance/movement games; and 5) playing musical instruments that require assorted bodily movements (Nocera, 1979). (*Ali Zadeh Mohammadi*)

developmental grid

An organizational structure for an individual child and/or group in therapy and special education (Goodman, 2007). The grid includes the respective names of children longitudinally and educational/therapeutic goals pertaining to four developmental areas (social–emotional, cognitive, speech–language, motor) horizontally. In this way, it is easier to see goal areas that overlap in the session as well as goal areas that are most germane to MT. (*Karen Goodman*)

developmental, individual-difference, relationship-based (DIR) model

Developed by Dr Stanley Greenspan (Greenspan and Weider, 1998), the developmental, individual-difference, relationship-based DIR Floortime model makes reference to core capacity building and six milestones that emphasize cognitive affective development in child development (Greenspan and Weider, 1998). Failure to thrive and master the milestones may be attributed to sensory and neurological differences that are addressed through intervention, most notably referred to as Floortime. The model was first contextualized in MT by Goodman (2007: 89–97) as appropriate for individual MT, particularly one-to-one with children on the autistic spectrum. Other *mts* have since adopted it and/or contextualized it within the Nordoff–Robbins model (Carpente, 2011). (*Karen Goodman*).

dialogical perspective of music as therapy

Rudy Garred (2006) proposes that, 'it is insufficient to state that change through music is purely a musical matter and that musical change in and of itself cannot be defined as therapeutic change' (Young, 2007). Informed by Buber's (1958) seminal text, *I and Thou*, Garred argued that, in a musical encounter, one can never entirely predict music's effects through our personal relationships with music, others, time, place and context. Dialogue, both musical and non-musical, can be a reciprocal and mutual process rather than the means to an end. Garred's theory is applicable to multiple MT methods (Ansdell, 2006). (*Kevin Kirkland*)

directed imagery with music

Also known as guided imagery and not to be confused with the Bonny Method of Guided Imagery and Music, this technique uses therapist-guided imagery with a therapeutic intention (directives) given to a client for purposes of relaxation, spirituality, physical health issues and other needs where structured guiding is a supportive and effective treatment intervention. Heal and Wigram (1993) say that careful consideration is needed in selecting music that supports the imagery, with considerations for the music being familiar or unfamiliar, programmatic, matching mood, grounding versus freeing and at a volume that allows it to be in the background, so that the therapist's voice can be in the foreground and audible. (*Kevin Kirkland*)

discussion techniques

Generally, the various ways that *mts* engage clients in verbal discussion in conjunction with MT processes. Bruscia (1987a) uses the term as one of eight categories of clinical improvisation techniques used by *mts*. Ten verbal techniques are defined in this context: connecting, probing, clarifying, summarizing, feedback, interpreting, metaprocessing, reinforcing, confronting and disclosing. (*Lillian Eyre*)

dissonance

Occurs when simultaneous musical sounds are perceived as inharmonious. Typically, dissonance creates a sense of tension or instability that is resolved when the music moves to a more pleasing harmony. The perception of dissonance depends in large part on musical acculturation; an interval that is considered dissonant in one music tradition may be considered harmonious in another. There is also considerable variation in the treatment of dissonance. Some music styles tend to avoid dissonance altogether, for example, while others use it freely without resolution and still others have rules for resolving dissonances in predictable ways. (*Catherine Schmidt-Jones*)

documentation

Davis, Gfeller, and Thaut (1999) say that 'the submission of regular and accurate written reports is a fundamental responsibility of music therapists' (p. 283). Documentation, typically maintained by those in private practice or where clinical settings require or benefit from comprehensive write-ups of the MT intervention process. Documentation should be music-centred; reflect assessment data; goals, objectives, interventions and plans; and demonstrate evidence of change or maintenance of abilities. Writing should be objective, clear, concise and suited to the practice setting. All record keeping needs to be mindful of content, privacy, confidentiality and safe storage. Codes of ethics may also inform documentation protocols. (*Kevin Kirkland*)

drone

A simple accompaniment in which the same pitch or pitches sound continuously or repeatedly for the entirety or a substantial portion of a musical piece. A drone may consist of a single pitch, a chord or even a dissonance. 'Open' intervals of an octave, fifth or fourth are particularly favoured in many traditions. A drone may be produced by any pitched instrument, including voice, but there are instruments that specialize in providing drones, such as the *tanpura* in Indian music and the bagpipes in Scottish music. By providing a stable, audible reference point, the drone creates a strong sense of a 'home' pitch in the music. It also interacts with more active melodic lines to create harmonies and dissonances. (*Catherine Schmidt-Jones*)

drum play

The use of percussion instruments for pre-musical, extra-musical and/or non-musical experience. The visual, tactile, and physical properties of instruments are a key focus of drum play. Musical outcomes are a secondary consideration (Das and Matney, 2011). (*Kalani Das*)

drumming

The act of creating rhythms or beats on a drum or other hard surface using sticks, mallets or one's hands and fingers. Drumming is a universal activity, used in many different cultures as a means of communication, relationship building and healing. As a result, drumming has many therapeutic applications. A basic drum beat can resemble a heartbeat, creating a sense of primacy that reaches all people, regardless of ability. Repetition and stability of the beat can achieve qualities of grounding and holding. Physical movements involved in drumming support an individual's range of motion and coordination and provide tactile stimulation. Non-verbal communication is established through call and response as well as rhythmic variability. When clients are able to establish entrainment through drumming, they may experience a sense of shared energy and community. Drumming is used in both individual and group settings by *mts* who are mindful of these possibilities. (*Shirley Khalil*)

dynamic batukada

Batukada (also spelled 'batucada') is a sub-style of samba and refers to an African-influenced, Brazilian percussive style involving a large variety of instruments. Dynamic batukada originated with Bar-Even and Pridor (2010), who integrate therapy with a dynamic application of musical instructions and instruments. Their co-lead model uses rhythm to achieve several personal and interpersonal goals related to sublimation, group rules versus freedom of expression, psychomotor skills, self-confidence and sense of belonging and nonverbal communication. Key elements of a dynamic batukada workshop are: the chaos phase, call and response, musical games and solo versus accompaniment. A main goal is to help clients to decrease anxiety by developing their ability to be in all of the phases and to move from one phase to another with joy and confidence. Dynamic batukada introduces the roles and meanings of the co-leaders: 'the guiding signal' and the 'grounding keeper', one of whom marks the transformation from phase to phase and the other who surveys the group and 'shows the way back home' (Bar-Even and Pridor, 2010). (*Roey Bar-Even and Shay Pridor*)

early interaction music therapy (EIMT)

May be seen as one part of baby science-based music therapies. EIMT is informed by infant development science, early interaction research, attachment patterns and treatment applications. EIMT is based on Stern's (1985a, 1985b) theory of vitality affects that serves as a framework for understanding infants' ways of experiencing and expressing themselves. Vitality affects are musical in nature and thus music may be an important tool for reaching and making contact during the earliest phases of human development (Ahonen-Eerikäinen, 1999). EIMT is sometimes based on solution-centred, supportive methods but usually is rooted in psychodynamically oriented methods concentrated on the primary caregiver's inner images of the infant (Carlsson, 2007) or primary attachment experiences of the caregiver (Lipponen, 2008). Treatment may also benefit from the implementation of early interaction assessment tools, such as the Care Index (Crittenden, 2007) or the Marshak Interaction Method (Marshak, 1960). One goal for EIMT is to find suitable dynamics, tempos and nuances for the primary caregiver's improvisation or mirroring of the infant to foster mutual contact, communication and enjoyment (Lipponen, 2008). EIMT may also involve elements of Theraplay (Booth and Jernberg, 2010), inviting the therapist to support the primary caregiver by offering care, structure and emotional support through music (Lipponen, 2005). (*Auli Lipponen*)

ecology

The modern concept of ecology was first developed within biology, where it refers to the reciprocal influences between organisms and their environments. Since the 1960s, the term has also been used as an influential metaphor in theories of human development. In the psychological literature, Bronfenbrenner's model of interacting systems has been especially influential. According to Bronfenbrenner (1979: 16–42), *microsystems* consist of the activities, roles and interpersonal relations experienced by the developing person in a given setting. *Mesosystems* refers to the interrelations between two or more systems in which the developing person actively participates, while *exosystems* refers to influential systems that do not involve the active participation of the developing person. *Macrosystems*, at the level of culture or society as a whole, frame the three lower-order systems. All human practices can be understood ecologically; changes at the level of the individual have implications for various social systems and vice versa. Bruscia (1998b) suggested the term 'ecological music therapy' to refer to practices where goals and interventions are centred on the fostering of health-promoting relationships between systems. In contemporary community MT theory, the ecological quality of practice is considered to be a key focal point (Stige and Aarø, 2012). (*Brynjulf Stige*)

educational music therapy

Defines the functional and scientific application of music by a trained mt to facilitate recall for educational purposes and to enhance transfer of information to non-musical settings (Silverman, 2007). Key components emphasized in the educational environment include the use of music as an information carrier or resource to aid memorization and listening to music or participating in different activities to maintain appropriate behavior and to support the completion of academic tasks. Educational MT offers social and emotional support to clients by using structured activities to practice different types of social behavior and to express emotion. MT supports music education because it offers different methods and techniques to ensure that students with learning disabilities participate successfully in the regular instructional environment (Davis, Gfeller, and Thaut, 2008). *(Ivana Ilic)*

ego strength

According to Wolberg (1977), 'ego strength' points to the positive personality assets that may enable the individual to overcome their anxieties and to acquire more sufficient defences. Success-oriented (failure-free) MT experiences can elicit improved mood and motivation in a framework where the client can trust their experiences. The client's ego develops and strengthens when the client is continually regarded through the therapist's empathic affirmations and through the musical relationship, where the *mt* identifies with the client's psychological reality (Wigram, Pedersen and Bonde, 2002b). MT has provided preliminary and promising evidence that could develop fundamental ego strength through enhancement of positive physical and psychological self-awareness and self-esteem (Wigram, Pedersen and Bonde, 2002a). (*Ali Zadeh Mohammadi*)

electronic music technology

May help to facilitate the successful manipulation of musical sounds by clients in different settings for different clinical purposes. Electronic resources, such as digital musical instruments and laptop or tablet computers, may be used by themselves or in conjunction with assistive technologies as needed by the client to operate and use these resources. *Assistive technology* refers to any piece of equipment or product system which is used to maintain or improve skills or capabilities of clients with disabilities (US Public Law 108–364: Assistive Technology Act of 2004). The many uses of electronic music technology to facilitate clinical MT success for clients with special needs have been detailed by a number of authors (Crowe and Rio, 2004; Krout, 2008; Magee and Burland, 2008). Assistive technologies may include: self-contained music-making/creating devices such as keyboards/synthesizers and drum/rhythm machines; electronic music devices used with a computer/other controller, including devices operated via MIDI (musical instrument digital interface); portable devices which operate music applications such as the iPad and other tablet computers; music composition, arranging, notation, improvisation and sequencing software; music recording modules; music playback and listening devices; and additional technologies, including music game-oriented systems. (*Robert Krout*)

embodiment

Emphasizes the bodily basis of mind, cognitive processes and cultural phenomena (Frank, 2007). Musical activities such as tapping to a beat and dancing and playing an instrument are not merely states resulting from mental processes. Rather, they can be conceived of as an initial state of a goal-directed process. Embodied views of music emphasize ways in which bodily activities participate in music perception, music-making and interpersonal communication. In neonate and infant MT, rhythmically coordinated synchronization between a lullaby sung by the caregiver and the infant's corporeal responses highlights the embodied and interactive nature of human musicality. (*Jin Hyun Kim*)

emotional processes in music therapy

Music can easily create access to a wide range of emotions. It can elicit or calm them. Emotional responses to music are highly individualized (Juslin *et al.*, 2010). In MT, emotions become audible, enabling the client to express, understand, work through, manage and accept them. This involves the non-verbal expression of emotions in a safe environment with the therapist containing and reflecting them. Vocal techniques can enhance emotional expression. Mary Priestley (1975) developed an emotional spectrum for mapping emotions that can be addressed in expressive analytical MT. She devised a 'seven main compound emotions model': freeze-fear, flight-fear, defensive-fear, anger, guilt, sorrow and love-joy-peace. In receptive MT music may become more emotionally charged than by usual (non-altered/alternate states of consciousness) music listening. Music is also found to be a prime evoker of peak experience (Whaley, Sloboda and Gabrielsson, 2008; Maslow, 1962). Transference and countertransference dynamics in MT may contain an emotional spectrum that can be processed nonverbally and/or verbally. Unique to the MT process is that the client can transfer a specific emotion or several emotions to one or more 'objects': a therapist, an instrument, the music and/or imagery evoked by music (Bruscia, 1998d). (*Alice Pehk*)

empathy

Refers to an interpersonal process of shared emotion unmediated by the rational mode of thinking. The original German term for empathy, *Einfühlung*, was used in the nineteenth century in the context of psychological aesthetics to describe an implicit and immediate process related to an aesthetic object (Lipps, 1903). Mechanisms of action–perception loops underlying empathy are investigated in current psychology and cognitive neuroscience in close relation to emotional contagion and motor mimicry. However, a process of the identification of self as distinguished from others is conceived of as central to empathy, whereas it is considered to be unnecessary for motor mimicry and emotional contagion. In MT, specific distinctions among empathy, motor mimicry, and emotional contagion have yet to be highlighted and decribed as key areas of research inquiry and practice. (*Jin Hyun Kim*)

empowerment

A concept used in resource-oriented MT (Rolvsjord, 2010), feminist MT (Curtis, 1996) and community MT (Procter, 2002). Rolvsjord (2010) describes three interdependent and interactive levels at which empowerment occurs: the individual, the organization and the community. Therapy that draws from empowerment philosophy focuses on client strengths and resources or potentials rather than weaknesses and pathologies. Emphasis is placed on egalitarian relationships and collaboration between therapist and client. In resource-oriented MT, empowerment is manifested through recognition of the client's competence, preference for ways of working and development of the client's resources: personal, social, economic and musical. Feminist approaches to MT acknowledge the interdependence of personal, interpersonal and institutional factors that impact on a client's health and wellbeing. Thus, empowerment is achieved by considering individual problems within wider social and institutional contexts, identifying and challenging conditions (external and internal) that are oppressive; and engaging the client's resources to work toward personal and social transformation. Likewise, in community MT, empowerment involves individual and collective changes within a cultural context. (*Susan Hadley*)

entrainment

The process of synchronization between two phenomena, such as the sympathetic vibration of one tuning fork with another of the same frequency; the bouncing of a bridge to regular footsteps; or the coordinated chirping of crickets. Entrainment was first described by Christiaan Huygens, the inventor of the pendulum clock in 1657, who noted that pendulums of the same length mounted on the same support become synchronized over time (Mannes, 2011: 21–22). In MT, the term refers to a coming together of music and client. Most commonly, this refers to heart-rate entrainment, so a tempo of a relaxed heart (MM = 60) is commonly used. Psychological entrainment between leader and group or client and therapist refers to matching energy level and speaking speed. Brainwave entrainment occurs through neural excitation resulting from regular music pulsation such as an arpeggio pattern, a fingerpicking pattern on a guitar or a xylophone mallet roll of a sustained pitch. Scientifically designed music may use specific sonic techniques to entrain (drive) brainwaves to boost a particular brain state. Entrainment also describes the cognitive process involved in mentally tracking the beat, anticipating the next occurrence and coordinating an action such as clapping with it. (*Lee Bartel*)

environmental music therapy

The use of live music to construct a soundscape which can modulate the perception of an existing environment. The soundscape is constructed in such a way as to reduce noise or incorporate ambient sounds as well as visual and aural cues from those present. Focus is placed on the conversion of disparate noxious stimuli often present in fragile environments into less threatening presences. Environmental music therapy is a term coined by Steve Schneider (Stewart and Schneider, 2000) and has been studied in applied research at Beth Israel Medical Center intensive care units in New York City. (*Joanne Loewy*)

epistemology

A branch of philosophy that studies the nature of knowledge (What is knowledge?), the foundations and presuppositions of knowledge (How is knowledge acquired?) and the limits and validity of knowledge (How do we know what we know?). In the field of epistemology, knowledge is analyzed in terms of how it relates to truth, belief and justification. In a positivist paradigm, knowledge is discovered and verified through direct observation and measurement. In a constructivist paradigm, knowledge is established through the meanings attached to that which is studied. While MT is grounded in an epistemological framework, epistemology is not widely studied in MT (Edwards, 2012). However, some researchers are arguing for the establishment of a theory of knowledge (epistemology) founded on musical experiences and our understandings and experiences as MT clinicians. Aigen (1991) states that, rather than forcing knowledge gained in the musical interactions of therapists and clients into categories derived from verbal traditions, we should create our own epistemology through musically obtained knowledge. In MT, Robbins and Forinash (1991) have explored this territory in terms of articulating a multilevel theory of time, one that was inspired by and demonstrated through specific MT experiences. (*Susan Hadley*)

ethics

A code of conduct guiding decision-making interactions between and among professionals, their clients, and the public. Dileo (2000) defines ethics or applied ethics as the beliefs and standards we adhere to regarding right and wrong behaviour in a professional encounter or setting. 'Professional ethics refers to the principles (both explicit and general) and expectations of conduct for members of a profession towards clients, peers, the public, and employers, and are based on specific responsibilities to these parties. These principles are expressed as guidelines and comprise the *Code of Ethics* for a profession' (p. 3). Adherence to ethical guidelines is especially important in health care when dealing with confidential material and power differentials between caregivers and those needing care, and when navigating relationships with other professionals. (*Robin Rio*)

ethnicity

Refers to a group of people who share a common heritage or ancestry, a common language, a common distinctive culture, common traditions involving food, clothing, beliefs, music and other elements, and historical memories. Ethnicity is often viewed as belonging to a minority group. Generally, those who do not define themselves in terms of ethnicity are in a dominant social group. However, even those belonging to the dominant culture have an ethnic identity. Ethnic identity may be heightened owing to migration or colonization. In some societies, social stratification is based on ethnicity, sometimes leading to interethnic conflict. In MT, ethnicity is largely explored and addressed through multicultural or culturally sensitive approaches. (*Susan Hadley*)

ethnography

A qualitative research method about a specific culture or way of life that seeks to understand a given culture in its own terms and often puts the researcher's way of life into perspective (Hammersley and Atkinson, 1983). Yehuda (2002) sees the research field as a social world. She refers to ethnography within MT stemming from Stige (2002a) who proposed clinical research as ethnography (culture-centred), Ruud (1980, 1998) and Aldridge (1999). (*Julie Lytle*)

eurythmy

Developed by Steiner in 1912, eurythmy is an art form and a concept of movement in which creative and formational powers of sound (speech or music) are made visible (Steiner, 1983; Ogletree, 1976: 305 ff). It differs from Dalcroze's eurythmics, which is a form of dance to melody. The eurythmist must first experience the formation and structure of musical sounds or a poem and only later bring them to eurythmic expression. Heirman (1971) said, 'the Eurythmist has to conduct all the motions of his body, which work together in their artistic development [and expression] as a soundless orchestra' (p. 15). (*Kevin Kirkland*)

evaluation

An analysis occurring periodically or at termination of MT to determine the success of treatment. Review of data that quantifies and qualifies client progress toward clinical goals and objectives is the form of evaluation in Hanser's (1999) data-based model of MT. Evaluation looks for evidence of change and is an opportunity for the *mt* to reflect upon interventions, methods applied, revisions and updates of goals and objectives and peer consultations. Client self-evaluation of progress and other subjective measures are used in various models of MT. (*Donna Chadwick*)

event segmentation

The engagement of the brain through music to make sense of the constant input and flow of information. 'The brain partitions information about beginnings, endings, and the boundaries between events' (Baker, 2007: 1). This could be a useful element in teaching boundaries to clients through the use of structured musical events. Since music engages the brain over time, musical processing may aid the brain in event anticipation through sustained attention. The implications for use of elements found in speech, such as phrasing, silence and contour, may translate into psychological and embodied ways of understanding and living in the world. (*Kevin Kirkland*)

everyday creativity

Richards (2010) defines this term of 'human originally at work and leisure across the diverse activities of everyday life' (p. 190). This type of creativity differs from eminent creativity, that which is novel and serves a function and also makes changes within a specific domain. Eminent creativity occurs in great artists, scientists and inventors, whereas everyday creativity is evenly distributed across the population and is necessary for the survival of the human species. MT examples include: engaging clients in song writing; improvising; adapting instruments for accessibility or novel use; negotiating relationship dynamics; and, generally, exploring and solving a variety of challenges and problems. Everyday creativity can have health benefits related to resilience. (*Paul Nolan*)

evidence-based mental health (EBMH)

Represents a qualitative shift in prescriptive views of health care to ones in which 'the psyche of the client is the centre of attention' (Smeijsters, 2006: 805). EBMH uses both client and therapist experienced-based knowledge integrated into best practices. Criteria to assess effectiveness may follow a qualitative paradigm of credibility, dependability (completeness of results), confirmability (outsider review), transferability (replication, similarities/differences in another context) and authenticity (participants contribute to meaning making) (Smeijsters, 2006). (*Kevin Kirkland*)

evidence-based music therapy practice

Evidence-based practice, as a general construct in health care, has been defined by the Agency for Healthcare Research and Quality (2009) as 'applying the best available research results (evidence) when making decisions about health care. Health care professionals who perform evidence-based practice use research evidence along with clinical expertise and client preferences. Systematic reviews (summaries of health care research results) provide information that aids in the process of evidence-based practice'. The AMTA (2010) has endorsed the following definition of evidence-based practice in the following way: 'Evidence-based music therapy practice integrates the best available research, the *mts*' expertise, and the needs, values, and preferences of the individual(s) served'. Abrams (2010) has provided the following definition of it, intended to support different understandings of evidence from objective, subjective, inter-objective and intersubjective perspectives: 'When client and therapist work together through music to promote health, guided by grounds sufficient to help ensure that the work is valuable' (p. 360). (*Brian Abrams*)

existential music therapy

'An optimistic approach that embraces human potential, while remaining a realistic approach through its recognition of human limitation' (Hoffman, 2004). Existential views of therapy are informed by understandings of meaning-making and psychopathology in the research literature. Yalom (1980) identifies psychopathology with four concerns related to maladaptive ways of coping: death, freedom/groundlessness, isolation, and meaninglessness (Yalom, 1980: 423, 482). Frankl (2004) in his discussion of meaninglessness, argues that existential neurosis (psychopathology) may develop when the will-to-meaning (the ability to make meaning that may develop out of suffering, doing a deed, or experiencing a value) is frustrated (Frankl, 2004: 88). MT supports engagement-in-life as the primary therapeutic answer to meaninglessness. Broucek (1987) views 'our task as a reviving of the life spirit... restoring a belief in the value of life [through the music therapy process]' (p. 39) Ruud (in Bohnert, 1999) said that 'music can provide a sense of community and intimacy with others' [thus creating meaning and breaking the isolation]' (p. 69). A creative experience that is highly meaningful for a client may aid in developing an individual's inner resources, reality-testing abilities and interpersonal communication, allowing for a stronger sense of presence in the here and now. (*Kevin Kirkland*)

experimental improvisation therapy

An improvisational model of MT developed by Riordan and Bruscia in 1972 (Bruscia, 1987b). Riordan originally conceived of experimental improvisation therapy as a method for using dance to help intellectually disabled adults develop creativity, self-expression and interpersonal skills. This improvisational dance model was adapted for MT by Bruscia to develop an interdisciplinary, improvisational model that could be implemented through dance, music or a combination of both. Issues of creativity, interpersonal freedom and responsibility were explored through group problem solving. *Experimental* denotes the improvisational method in which certain variables are held constant while others are systematically manipulated or allowed to vary freely. Three components are applied to help the group find a focus for exploration: vocabulary, procedures and relationships. The second cycle uses rehearsing, reconnecting and reacting (Bruscia, 1987b). (*Lillian Eyre*)

external validation

When they are in a group home, hospital or rehabilitation centre, clients often feel cut off from, and and, in some cases, looked down upon, by the outside world. External forms of validation may help to improve individual and group affect. Clients' sense of self-worth and connection to a group may improve when they are given awards and have opportunities to showcase their talents in person and for publications. At Queen's Park Health Care Center in New Westminster, British Columbia, Canada, a musical instrument-making group was awarded thousands of dollars by the Queen's Park Healthcare Foundation (http://qphf.org) and was pictured and written up in a catalogue distributed all over North America. In addition, a local newspaper sent a professional photographer to the facility and published an article about the residents and the instruments they had made. Staff and family members who viewed instruments being made saw clients in a new light. Not only did clients feel a sense of accomplishment but they also had something meaningful to discuss. (*Jeremie Tucker*)

family music therapy

Family members of an MT client with special needs, play a key role in the treatment process, building and strengthening connections among the client, therapist, music, and themselves. Family members often know a client better than an *mt* and can provide valuable information about a client's needs, emotions, gestures, words and sounds. Information about the effects of music on a client may also be shared and described by family members outside an MT session. It is important for *mts* to recognize that the family, as well as the client, has a vested interest in therapy and that, therefore, the group as whole benefits from active participation in the treatment process. (*Gabriel Federico and Brenda Woldman*)

feminist music therapy

An approach first coined by Sandra Curtis in the late 1990s while developing her own feminist MT practice and given further attention in Hadley's (2006) book. Ideally, feminist MT is gender-balanced rather than androcentric or gender-centric; multicultural rather than ethnocentric or heterosexist; focuses on social interactions rather than intra-psychic concepts; and is lifespan-oriented. Making an important shift away from a symptom-based approach, feminist music therapy emphasizes resilience, empowerment and a resource-oriented paradigm (Rolvsjord, 2010). It strives for non-hierarchical, egalitarian interpersonal relationships, including the therapeutic relationship, and employs practices of demystification; that is, transparency about the therapeutic process. FMT also engages in feminist-informed analyses of power and analyses of gender-role socialization and works toward social transformation. Feminist music therapy is a consciousness-raising approach that focuses on the heterogeneous reality of women's as well as men's personal and social identities. Feminist *mts* stress the significance of understanding the social premises of music and challenging the social functions of MT that unconsciously perpetuate gender oppression and other oppressions. (*Susan Hadley*)

first-person action research

Any method in which the researchers or participants gather data from themselves, using processes such as introspection, retrospection or self-studies. Applications of first-person action research include self-inquiry (Roberts, 2003), autoethnography and autobiography. The therapist-as-subject engages experience reflexively in relationship to MT practice and personal and professional development. Roberts (2008) says that the value of the method is that it aids in understanding the pioneering of a new type of practice, to represent learning moments, to link personal learning to scholarship and to improve the researcher's own practice. Qualitative data are gathered through a predetermined lens and then later analyzed and reflected upon; the results sometimes creatively cast for sharing. (*Kevin Kirkland*)

flow

A psychological term first used by Hungarian psychologist Mihaly Csikszentmihalyi (1991) to describe a state of total focus and concentration. When in a flow state, a person is operating at peak arousal and ability, and is experiencing enjoyment from the activity. Individuals who are in a flow state are often unaware of the passage of time, their physiological needs or their surroundings (if their surroundings are not important to the task they are performing). Flow states can occur during almost any activity and are particularly evident during musical performances, especially those involving improvisation (Bengtsson, 2007). Flow states are often colloquially described by such expressions as 'in the zone' and 'in the moment'. (*Charles Limb and Malinda McPherson*)

focal music therapy in obstetrics (FMTO)

Developed by Dr Héctor J. Fiorini, Professor of Psychoanalytic Psychotherapies in the School of Psychology, University of Buenos Aires, Argentina in 1991, this model is intended for pregnant women and/or their partners. "It is known as Focal Music Therapy Focused on Obstetrics for two main reasons: The first one is the brief duration of treatments, and the second is the focal concept (developed by Dr. Fiorini) this type of therapy is carried out with" (Federico, 2005: 1). Therapy addresses the overlapping physical, mental, emotional, and spiritual 'spheres' of pregnancy; when these are out of balance, *mts* work on 'tuning' them to assist a well-balanced pregnancy. There are seven key processes associated with FMTO: 1) relaxation through movement, 2) a welcome song, 3) creative visualization with music, 4) prenatal musical stimulation, 5) vibrational massage, 6) sound bath, and 7) directed improvisation with musical instruments (Federico, 2011: 1). One or more processes may be used during the therapy session, depending on a client's needs and the skills of the *mt*. FMTO seeks to improve the quality of a woman's pregnancy; stimulate and strengthen early bonding among mother, father, and baby, and improve the baby's quality of life in pre-, peri-, and post-natal stages (Federico, 2005: 2–3). (*Gabriel Federico*)

free association during free improvisation

A process wherein the client is encouraged to verbally free associate thoughts, feelings, phrases and sounds that spontaneously arise to a titled or untitled free improvisation. The process, informed by Nachmanovitch (1990) is extended into the addition of vocalizations/verbalizations, potentially stimulating the improvisation into depth process or alternate territory, offering an opportunity for unconscious or preconscious material to surface and be externalized when given voice, shape, sound and meaning. (*Kevin Kirkland*)

free associative singing

A technique within vocal psychotherapy (Austin, 2009) that can be implemented when words enter the vocal holding process. Clients are encouraged to sing any words that occur to them while the two-chord holding pattern accompaniment and the therapist's singing continue to contain the client's process. The emphasis, however, is not only on 'holding' the client's emerging self and psychic contents but also on creating momentum through the music and the lyrics that will propel the improvisation and therapeutic process forward. Throughout the improvisation, the therapist is making critical decisions about when, how and what to sing with the client. With the movement to words from vocalizations, there is often a need for variations in the music to reflect changes in the client's feelings. (*Diane Austin*)

free group sound association

In the context of an analytic MT group, wherein the spontaneous musical improvisation of the members is a predominant medium, Foulkes' (1968/1990) free group association assumes the form of free group sound association (Agrotou, 1998). Any sound created by a group member is considered a free group sound association. This is derived from Foulkes' concept of free group association characterizing the analytic group. The spontaneous responses of each member, as they follow one another, bear an unconscious interconnection and entail an interpretation to what has been said before in the group. This free group association is based on the common ground of unconscious instinctive understanding that the members share within the group matrix (Foulkes, 1968/1990). It is not only the verbal content that is associative in this way but also the form of speech, its expressive qualities, the 'silences and other non-verbal communications, facial and other expressions, appearance, attitudes, gestures, actions' (ibid: 180). In an analytic MT group each member's sound expression, even when it occurs simultaneously to the sounds of others, is a meaningful reaction – a resonance or a contradiction, a confirmation or a denial, an elaboration or a synopsis – to what another is currently, or has just, expressed. (*Anthi Agrotou*)

free improvisation

Wigram and De Backer (1999: 117–18) say that free improvisation is spontaneous and involves playing an instrument with minimal prior instruction. The improvisation process typically begins with the client choosing an instrument for musical expression supported musically by the *mt*. Wigram and De Backer point out that the musical interventions and responses of the *mt* influence the direction of the music. Many improvisational models of MT involve free improvisation and serve as a basis of uncovering interaction styles, emotions, patterns, personality and relationship with/to music. (*Kevin Kirkland*)

free improvisation therapy

A developmental approach in which musical instruments are of central importance to the client–therapist relationship. Developed by Juliette Alvin (1975), this method was described by Bruscia (1987c) as free improvisation therapy. In it, the therapist gives the client complete freedom to improvise as they wish, without any rules, structures or themes. Alvin identified three developmental stages to her approach: Association, Identification, Integration. 1) Sound exploration (instrument=Association); 2) Dyadic improvisation (*mt*=Identification); 3) Group improvisation (others=Integration). Two major models of improvisational MT are: 1) analytical music therapy (AMT) based on Priestley (1994); and 2) Creative Music Therapy (CMT), developed by Nordoff and Robbins (1977). In AMT, the client and therapist identify an issue through verbal discussion. After the roles of the two participants are defined, this issue serves as a title or theme for improvisation. In CMT, improvisations are non-referential. Therapist and client co-create music without giving titles to, and without discussing the music. This approach is essential for children and other clients whose verbal means of expression is extremely limited or non-existent (Pavlicevic, Trevarthen, and Duncan, 1994). (*Ali Zadeh Mohammadi and Debbie Carroll*)

free play

Improvisation without rules of play or preconceived associations or references from either client or therapist. Free play can provide a sense of freedom by honouring the client's music. Free play may be contraindicated for those who benefit from structure and context, such as clients for whom anxiety may be overwhelming and rules and boundaries would be a preferred starting place to experience improvisation. Through spontaneous expression, creativity is awakened and one's authentic self and voice can emerge (Nachmanovitch, 1990). (*Shirley Khalil*)

Gaston, E. Thayer (1901–1970)

Everett Thayer Gaston was a psychologist often referred to as the 'father' of MT in the USA, where he worked at the University of Kansas as Professor of Music Education and Director of Music Therapy. He proposed eight seminal ideas about MT: 1) all humans need aesthetic expression and experience; 2) the cultural matrix determines the mode of expression; 3) music and religion are integrally related; 4) music is communication; 5) music is structured reality; 6) music is derived from tender emotions; 7) music is a source of gratification; 8) the potency of music is greatest in the group (Gaston, 1968). While chair of the music education department at the University of Kansas, Gaston received encouragement from doctors at the Menninger Foundation in Topeka, Kansas, for his ideas regarding the use of music as an adjunctive therapy for the mentally ill. He then established the first graduate degree programme in the USA for MT training. 'His insatiable thirst for knowledge, dedication to scholarship, and unquestioned integrity led to his preeminent position in this field' (Johnson, 1981). (*Kevin Kirkland*)

gay affirmative therapy (GAT)

The term 'gay affirmative' was coined by clinical psychologist Alan Malyon (1982) in an article defining GAT. It emphasizes an affirming, non-pathological view of therapy with and for lesbian, gay and bisexual (LGB) persons. Developed in the 1970s and 1980s, it was the first therapeutic movement that acknowledged harm done to LGB individuals through heterosexist socialization and institutional homophobia (Lev, 2005). GAT serves to: 1) counter negative sociocultural and familial environments of LGB clients; 2) address the negative effects of growing up in an oppressive society; and 3) facilitate the coming-out process and the development of a positive LGB identity (Milton and Coyle, 2002). GAT has been refined and adapted by many therapists, and is currently viewed as an approach rather than a theoretical model of psychotherapy (Davies, 1996). This approach highlights the *mt*'s understanding of unique challenges facing LGB clients (Garnets and Kimmel, 2003); introduces possibilities for resolving one's heterosexist prejudices and homophobia (Harrison, 2000); and familiarizes therapists with models of sexual identity development (Davies, 1996) and LGB culture and society (Milton and Coyle, 1999). (*Bill Ahessy*)

gender

Historically, gender referred to distinguishing characteristics between males and females, particularly in the cases of men and women, and the masculine and feminine attributes assigned to them, from physiological characteristics to social roles and gender identities. Concurrently, the term was often used euphemistically to avoid the word 'sex'. In diverse modern cultures, gender is increasingly applied to social contexts, while 'sex' is applied to physiological distinctions. In addition, there is increased understanding that there are not two, male/female, either/or genders, but rather, there are 'shades of difference' (Fausto-Sterling, 2000: 3). Previous rigid social distinctions of gender have started shifting based on liberalization of societal norms. Persons express their gender identities based on a sense of individual inner drives, desires and understandings in what continues to be a gender-structured society. Bill Ahessy (2011) noted that, although the published field of MT has addressed many areas of societal inequities through multiculturalism, the area of gender discrimination and, particular to his paper, issues of sexual orientation need to be clearly integrated into training programmes to ensure best practice care for all. (*Sue Baines*)

genogram

A visual representation of family history and relationships spanning at least three generations. Beyond the standard genealogical information of a family tree or anthropological kinship diagram, genograms include details regarding the emotional nature of relationships among family members; provide insight into the strengths, vulnerabilities and resources of families; and track the occurrence of patterns over time and across generations. Rooted in family systems theory, the understanding of the family culture that genograms foster is especially useful in cross-cultural work (Muchnik, 2006). Within therapy, genograms may be created by the therapist as a form of assessment or by clients as a means to increase awareness of their own family dynamics. In *Case Studies in Music Therapy* (LeFebvre, 1991), there is reference to an *mt* using a client-created, musical genogram to document musical histories of the client's family members. Bargiel (2004) suggested using musical genograms to assess parents' relationship to music when doing an MT intervention of parental singing for at-risk infants. Some *mts* have included sections for genograms on assessment forms. (*Julie Lytle*)

goals

The desired outcome of an MT treatment intervention. Goals are often broad and long-term, although they may also be single-session specific, depending on the setting. Goals can be drawn from and refer to various domains, including social, emotional, behavioural, cognitive, spiritual, communication and/or motor domains. An example of a goal within the cognitive domain might be for the client to improve decision making. (*Cynthia Colwell*)

goodbye song

Typically, the final song of an MT session. It may be pre-composed or improvised, depending on the style of therapy being delivered. The goodbye song is used to provide closure for the session and is typically the same song every session to provide a ritualized context. (*Naomi Bell*)

grammar

Every language has its grammar, as does music, with its detailed rules governing the use of its melodic and harmonic signs. What was not allowed linguistically some time ago may now be viewed as acceptable. Rules of grammar, much like rules of music (such as music theory rules about four-part music not having consecutive fifths or octaves) change over time (Farnsworth, 1958: 85). Lerdahl and Jackendoff's (1983) theory of musical representation is partly founded on the basis that tonal music is constructed according to a rule-based grammar or syntax. Concepts from linguistics are used as an analytical framework in which musical grammar is viewed as having sets of explicit and implicit rules that determine how listeners experience the well-formedness of musical sequences (Sloboda, 2005). (*Kevin Kirkland*)

graphic notation

A method of representing musical structures or receptive music experiences in a visible form without exactly defined parameters and values. It can be used to make fast sketches for memorizing clinical improvisations; as a presentation format when *mts* present clinical material to other professionals; or as elaborated 'scores' for in-depth analysis of events or episodes within improvised or composed music. Graphic notation involves description of musical syntax as well as semantics. Bergstrøm-Nielsen (2010) has written extensively on its applicability to MT, and also internationally his ideas have been expanded (Cohen, Gilboa, Bergstrøm-Nielsen, Leder and Milstein 2012). (*Lars Ole Bonde*)

Greek modes

Before the modern-day modes known as the major and minor scales or keys, there were many other modes in regular use (Farnsworth, 1958: 281). Naturally, there are multiple variations of both modes and scales from around the world. Greek modes come in at least seven varieties according to second-century musician and astronomer Ptolemy (Craig, 2012), although their exact uses and health benefits remain blurry, as does the formula of how the modes changed over time. There are vast differences between ancient Greek modes and their later interpretations and applications in the Middle Ages. Ptolemy lists the Greek modes as: Dorian on D (all white notes), Phrygian on F♯, Lydian on G♯, Mixolydian on B, Hypophyrian on C♯, and Hypolydian on D♯. These modern modes of the Middle Ages can be expressed using only the white notes on a piano, starting on a different pitch. Commonly accepted modes are: Dorian on D, Phrygian on E, Lydian on F, Mixolydian on G, Hypodorian (or Aeolian) on A, Hypophrygian or Locrian on B and Hypolydian (later known as Ionian) on C (Ball, 2010). Modes can be conducive to accessing alternate moods and states of consciousness through their unfamiliarity to contemporary scales. (*Kevin Kirkland*)

grounded theory

A qualitative research approach focused on generating theory about a phenomenon under study (Corbin and Strauss, 2007; Glaser and Strauss, 2009). Researchers gather data from a variety of sources, including interviews, field observations, videotape reviews, and reflexive journals. They analyze data using inductive strategies, such as coding, then organize results into emerging themes and categories. During the data analysis, grounded theory researchers attempt to derive meaning and interpret the data avoiding *a priori* assumptions and research hypotheses. According to Amir (2005), most *mts* have used modified grounded theory research methodology because of the difficulty in describing the psychological processes involved in studying MT phenomena without applying pre-existing knowledge. (*Varvara Pasiali*)

group analytical music therapy

Informed by the work of group analysts such as Bion and, predominantly, S. H. Foulkes (Woodcock, 1987). Clients who meet in the context of a group-analytic situation create a shared psychic life wherein mental aspects of their personalities interact instinctively and basically unconsciously. This is the group's *foundation matrix*; as relationships become more intimate, the members form a constantly developing *dynamic matrix* (Foulkes, 1973/1990). *Matrix* means a psychic network of communication in which the individuals are the nodal points, producing the network and at the same time being permeated by it (Foulkes, 1968/1990). Whatever an individual expresses concerns the whole group and finds some immediate resonance in other members, who respond to it according to their own level of functioning. In similar ways, in group analytic music therapy, any spontaneous sound, verbal or non-verbal expression, is considered to be a meaningful link between group members, through which transferences are expressed and unconscious levels of the group matrix are explored (Towse, 1997; Ahonen-Eerikäinen, 2007). The group therapist neither leads nor creates the group's ideas, but directs the procedure, fostering group culture through stances and interventions used. (*Anthi Agrotou*)

group improvisational music therapy

A five-segment session format originally created by Burns while working with oncology patients in a group setting. The segments, informed by humanistic values, are: 1) welcome (group members are encouraged to individually share and express their immediate feelings either verbally or non-verbally); 2) group awareness (the group is invited to choose instruments to accompany the therapist in improvisation if and when clients feel comfortable doing so, encouraging them to become aware of each other's playing); 3) exploration of emotions (the group decides on goals to be pursued during session and the type of improvisation it wishes to create to explore emotions. Improvisations may be either themed or non-themed); 4) relaxation and reflection (the therapist plays instrument of the group's choice while clients relax and reflect upon their own created improvisations); and 5) verbal processing and closure (the group is encouraged to share and process thoughts, feelings and/or insights gained during relaxation and reflection leading to closure). (*Sarah Burns*)

Guided Imagery and Music, Bonny Method of (GIM)

GIM was developed by Dr Helen Bonny (1978/2002, 1999a, 1999b, 2002) in the early 1970s based upon her prior work at the Maryland Psychiatric Research Center, where she combined relaxation techniques and classical music selections to support clients undergoing LSD-assisted psychotherapy. Defined as 'A music-centered exploration of consciousness that uses specifically sequenced classical music programs to stimulate and sustain a dynamic unfolding of inner experiences, offering persons many possibilities for wholeness. Among the fundamental tenets of this method are: the acceptance of both imagery and music as therapeutic agents; the acknowledgement of both transpersonal and psychodynamic aspects of the therapeutic journey; and the search to understand the therapeutic significance of expanded awareness experiences' (Association for Music and Imagery, 2011). GIM is practiced internationally, primarily in a variety of psychotherapy and counselling settings. (*Brian Abrams*)

guided interactive drumming

A directive, highly structured drumming experience where clients (participants) base their musical participation on rules, instruction and cues as provided by the therapist (leader). Guided interactive drumming may take the form of a 'game' or may incorporate formal musical structures as a foundation for guided play. (*Kalani Das*)

hand-over-hand

A form of gestural cue used for encouraging or modelling appropriate or desired behaviours and/or expectations during an MT session. Therapists may use hand-over-hand cues to: a) encourage a client to start or stop playing; b) assist a client in holding musical instruments (e.g. mallets, non-pitched percussion); c) teach a specific music skill (e.g. a rhythmic or melodic pattern, a chord); or d) prompt a specific communicative response (e.g. identifying a picture by pointing or reaching for an instrument). The *mt* may gradually fade use of hand-over-hand cues when working towards more subtle prompts. (*Varvara Pasiali*)

harmonics

Component frequencies of vibrating media, such as strings, plates, membranes and air columns. Harmonics are integer multiples of the fundamental frequency of a pitch and are often heard in combinations above that pitch as overtones (1/2, 1/3, 1/4, etc.). The fundamental frequency of a pitch (e.g. 440 Hertz) is called the first harmonic, as it is an integer component (1/1) of the frequency. While a pure sine wave does not produce or include overtones, richer-sounding waves such as sawtooth or ramp waves include the fundamental frequency and overtones in decreasing amplitudes. These overtones and the resulting wave forms (e.g. sawtooth, square) may give an instrument a characteristic sound, as an instrument's timbre is partly determined by the harmonics produced when played. Certain MT techniques, such as chanting, toning and the use of sounding and singing bowls, may make use of harmonics as a unique part of the therapeutic sound environment and process. (*Robert Krout*)

harmony

The paired or chordal (three notes or more) organization of tones sounded together, usually consonant in nature (Ratner, 1966). MT helps clients to be connected through the use of harmony, which can help them to experience empathy that increases social bonds in a group or the therapeutic alliance when working one-to-one. Some *mts* develop the skill of providing a clear harmonic support instrumentally and/or vocally to a client's musical expression (Sloboda, 1991), which may be viewed as an extension of Priestley's 'holding' technique, as grounding and enriching the client's sound through the harmonic metaphor of being with the client but not on the same path note for note. (*Ali Zadeh Mohammadi*)

Haus, Reiner (b. 1962)

Dr Reiner Haus (Dr rer. medic.) is Director of the Music Therapy Department at Children's Hospital in Datteln (Veristische Kinder- und Jugendklinik Datteln, Universität Witten/Herdecke) in Germany. He founded the MT Masters programme at the University of Liepaja in Latvia (which he chaired from 2002–2006). In 2008, Dr Reiner received the 'best practice model' award from the German Council for Disability for his foundational work in MT services and research in Latvia. As a scientific advisor, he supports the academic, research and financial development of MT in Latvia. (*Mirdza Paipare*)

health musicking

Researchers continue to investigate the practices of expressive singing and playing and concentrated listening to music, as well as their influences on health; this confluence of salutary musical engagement is often referred to as 'health musicking', based on the concept of 'musicking' (Small, 1998), describing any form of participation in musical activities. Brynjulf Stige (2002a, 2003, 2012) first defined this term. Some now view the pursuit and maintenance of health as a bodily, creative and aesthetic act – even a 'health performance' – and music can offer many affordances and appropriations in this context (Bonde, 2011). Factors involved in health musicking include: 1) personal resources; 2) musical elements; and 3) various contextual aspects. (*Lars Ole Bonde*)

heart rate entrainment (HRE)

The phenomenon of the heart slowing its pulse when the client listens to music with a beat slower than the heart rate. With the influence of Georgi Lozanov's (1971) 'Super Learning' programme, slow movements from baroque compositions (with a typical MM of 60) were seen as the standard for slowing heart rate. Other music has been shown to have a similar effect. Rarely is there an actual 'phase locking' between beat and heart rate. Rather, music slower than the heart rate is heard as relaxing and the relaxation response slows the heart rate. Cognitive tracking of the beat does create a brain response (Fujioka *et al.*, 2009) that may affect heart rate. Cognitive tracking is made conscious with coordination of rhythmic breathing to the beat and consequently enhanced heart rate entrainment. (*Lee Bartel*)

heart rate variability (HRV)

Heart rate, commonly thought to be fairly steady on a moment-to-moment basis, actually fluctuates constantly as a function of the antagonistic relationship of the sympathetic and parasympathetic nervous systems. The measure of the varying interval between heartbeats is HRV and is of interest in MT (Iwanaga and Kobayashi, 2005), music medicine (Riganello *et al.,* 2010) and performance science (Wasley, Williamon and Taylor, 2011) as an indicator of emotional arousal and stress. HRV is analyzed in terms of power spectral density; specifically, the components of low frequency, high frequency and their ratios. In MT, it is important to note that a healthy, unstressed heart produces greater HRV. Decreased HRV has been shown to be an important predictor of higher mortality risk among selected adults, particularly those after acute myocardial infarction (Cripps *et al.,* 1991; Quintana *et al.,* 1997). Although HRV may be a useful research tool, its place in clinical medicine and MT requires further investigation. Specific uses of music for increasing HRV may play critical roles in the future of cardiac therapy. (*Lee Bartel and David Alter*)

Heimlich model see paraverbal therapy

hello song

Helps clients with the concept of beginnings and can serve in a similar capacity to the contact song. The client's name can be used in a song to personalize the experience and to strengthen their identity. The day of the week or time of day or season can also be mentioned in the song to provide familiarity from week to week, an anchor in time. (*Monique van Bruggen-Rufi*)

Hello Space© model

Canadian *mt* Susan Summers developed this psychospiritual model (Summers, 1999), originally for older adults in residential long-term care settings but appropriate for clients in other settings. As *mts,* we say hello and we sing hello as a way of greeting and assessing a client's current state, and to initiate therapeutic connection. The Hello Space model takes this social and therapeutic hello to a deeper, more intimate level, acknowledging the inner and eternal within the person, by connecting and forming relationship with another human being. Saying hello to a client connects the *mt* with the well and whole part of the client, despite external, physical, spiritual, emotional and/or mental challenges. The model has four components: hello is given from the *mt* with their self, the client, the music and the creative space. At the centre of the model is the *mt,* who gives and receives a hello with their self as therapist and as person. Mutual and reciprocal hellos are given and received from therapist to the client, in addition to the music that is being offered, played and sung, and also with the overall ambiance of the session, which is called the creative space. (*Susan Summers*)

Herman, Frances Korson (b. 1927)

In the 1950s, Fran Herman became a pioneer of MT in Canada when she founded 'The Wheelchair Players', a production company of young people with severe disabilities who created and performed wheelchair ballets and dramas. Throughout her career, Fran advocated for children with special needs, emphasizing their ability to be empowered through music and other creative arts. She became head of the creative arts therapies department at Hugh MacMillan Rehabilitation Centre and co-authored two books: *Creatability* (Herman and Smith, 1992) and *Accentuate the Positive* (Herman and Smith, 1988). She was instrumental in the development of the Canadian MT profession, serving as the president of both the Ontario and Canadian associations. She helped to organize four national conferences, including the joint conference between the Canadian and American associations in 1993. In 1994, Fran became the first chair of the Canadian Music Therapy Trust Fund (http://www.musictherapytrust.ca) and with the help of her husband, Carl, raised over four million dollars for MT in Canada through the support of the recording industry. In 2002, she opened the Music Therapy Centre in Toronto. Fran has received many honours for her work, including the inaugural Music Advocacy Award of the Canadian Music Industry Association. (*Wanda Gascho-White*)

heuristic model of music therapy

Hillecke and Wilker (2007) and Hillecke, Nickel, and Bolay (2005) have summarized the therapeutic effects of MT in a heuristic model consisting of five working factors: 1) the modulation of attention (attention span and focus on assorted thoughts, feelings, images; 2) the modulation of emotions (associations and emotions triggered by music); 3) the modulation of cognition (reminders of past events, associations, conflicts, creative thinking); 4) the modulation of motor function and behaviour (music stimulus to condition behavioural patterns or rhythmic stimulation for entrainment in motor skills); 5) the modulation of communication (nonverbal communication, interpersonal events). A heuristic reading of MT may reveal 'hidden' truths about the MT process (Kirkland, 2004). It may also guide inquiry by offering a general formulation on music's therapeutic effects. (*Kevin Kirkland*)

hip-hop as therapy

A culturally sensitive and community-defined strategy that aims to enhance mental health. It has been used in therapy since the 1980s by *mts*, psychologists, social workers, dance/movement therapists, and poetry therapists (Tyson, 2002). This modality encompasses various aspects of hip-hop, a fluid and dynamic cultural site that consists of its own signature music, dance, art, dress, film, language, literature and social critique. Within the therapeutic context, hip-hop-as-therapy is not limited to the use of rap. Rather, it serves as an important cultural medium through which clients can incorporate a variety of creative hip-hop styles of expression and performance. These styles encourage powerful ways of performing and developing one's identity and finding value in one's creative potential and self-empowerment, through cathartic outlets such as graffiti art, break-dancing, lyric analysis, lyric writing and the creation of rap music (Hadley and Yancy, 2011). (*Susan Hadley*)

hippocampus

Part of the forebrain in the medial temporal lobe, it is critical in memory formation. It has a highly specialized cellular architecture consisting of two interlocking C-shaped strips of cortex, the dentate gyrus and the hippocampus proper. The hippocampus proper consists of four cornu ammonis (CA) fields. Information from a wide array of cortical neurons is funnelled into the granules cells of the dentate gyrus and then into the CA pyramidal cells. Outflow of the hippocampus is mainly from the pyramidal CA1 cells and subiculum. Damage or loss of neurons in the hippocampus can lead to impaired memory formation and susceptibility to seizures. According to Gaidos (2010), the hippocampus it known to play a role in long-term memory. It may help the brain to retrieve memories that give a sound meaning or context. It also aids linkage of previously heard music to an experience or context. The hippocampus and amygdala, which can both register strong emotions such as anxiety, are quieter during free improvisation (Miller, 2009). (*Robin Hsiung and Kevin Kirkland*)

holding

A concept developed by Winnicott (1960a, 1960b) to describe an important aspect of maternal provision: her ability in the first months of life to identify herself with her infant and therefore know what the infant feels and needs at any given moment. This enables her to 'hold' her infant in a way that provides security, stability and full adaptation to physiological and psychological needs. It includes 'especially the physical holding of the infant, which is a form of loving' (Winnicott, 1960b: 49). Translated into a therapeutic stance and technique, holding refers to the therapist's empathic understanding, correct and well-timed interpretation and supportive continuity (Winnicott, 1965). MT can offer a unique form of holding, as sounds, from vibration, are experienced as embracing the whole body. This offers a metaphor of Winnicott's physical holding. Thus, holding has been widely used by different MT approaches, often combined with containment. As such, it was first defined by Priestley (1975) as an analytical MT technique, followed by Bruscia, who described it as the therapist's sympathetic, background musical structure, which reverberates and contains the patient's feelings and 'provides a point of reference rather than an organizing or grounding force' (Bruscia, 1987a: 552). (*Anthi Agrotou*)

holding and reorganizing treatment modality

A method developed by Inge Nygaard Pedersen (1999) used in adult inpatient psychiatric settings to treat clients who have difficulty relating to others. The root of psychopathology here is viewed as possibly stemming from childhood dysfunction or trauma that is perpetuated throughout life as a learned behavioural pattern. Holding is a term borrowed from Winnicott (1960a, 1960b) and Priestley's (1975) approach and here is based on the theory of repairing an early disconnection or lack of symbiosis with the adult primary caregiver, typically the mother. The *mt* takes the premise that the client can reorganize the ability to be in relationship with another with the aim of breaking the isolation and forming a therapeutic alliance. The emphasis is on here-and-now processing rather than reliving and re-experiencing earlier traumatic events. Personal development is seen as possible by working through the 'cyclic dynamic understanding' of psychological problems (Nygaard Pedersen, 1999: 26–28). (*Kevin Kirkland*)

holding environment

A term developed by paediatrician and psychoanalyst D. W. Winnicott to describe 'the natural skill and constancy of care of the *good enough mother*' (or a primary caregiver) (Moore and Fine, 1990: 205). This allows the infant to experience omnipotence as an essential and regular feature of child development. The security afforded the infant provides for crucial preparation for later phases of development and separation. In MT, the concept of a holding environment can be demonstrated metaphorically via the therapist's support for the client, the boundaries of regularly scheduled sessions, similarities of events across sessions, empathy and uses of music for relaxation to help contain changes in emotional states that may arise during therapy. (*Paul Nolan*)

home-based music therapy (HBMT)

Allows for long-term (e.g. traumatic brain injury, chronic illness, dementia) or short-term (e.g. palliative care) community approaches to treatment (Schmid and Ostermann, 2010). Horne-Thompson (2003) compared therapist roles between institutional sites and home-based care and found that HBMT is influenced by four factors: 1) the client's will to participate is determined by the way the MT is introduced; 2) the role of the MT varies greatly between home and a hospital; 3) session length is potentially longer at home; 4) HBMT allows more opportunities for presence of other caregivers and their participation. (*Kevin Kirkland*)

human rights

The core set of rights enshrined in international law on behalf of all persons, regardless of race, colour, sex, sexuality, language, religion, political or other opinion, national or social origin, property, birth or other status (Clarke, 2010).

Some consider that human rights evolved out of these components: 1) civil and political rights; 2) economic, social and cultural rights; and 3) solidarity rights (Goodale, 2009). Freedom rights include freedom of speech, the press, religion, assembly and association (Abukishek, 2011). In recent years, *mts* have become increasingly involved in reaching out to survivors of war and related forms of violence. Some have been actively using music and/or MT to work towards their vision of peace, including the Music Therapists for Peace organization (Boxill, 1988). These practices are relevant to the world given the international nature of terrorism in this post-9/11 world. Music making draws out the essential humanity of the most unreachable people and places it in direct opposition to political violence, which denies the humanity and individuality of its victim. Music reflects positive anti-oppressive truths for many people and expresses love, kindness, tenderness and human rights (Dixon, 2002). People have the potential to express themselves through the development of creative interaction in a sound experience of understanding, love, intimacy and peace (Zadeh Mohammadi, 2002). (*Ali Zadeh Mohammadi*)

humanistic (person-centred) music therapy (HMT)

A theoretical and practical orientation to MT based largely upon principles of humanistic psychology, described by theorists such as Rogers (1951, 1961, 1980) and Maslow (1954, 1962). These principles assert that health consists of attributes of being such as a sense of personal identity, mobilization of autonomy and self-determination, creation of life meaning and purpose, establishment of basic dignity, cultivation of self-esteem, pursuit of personal values, fulfilment of individual potential and self-actualization. HMT provides opportunities for self-development and improved health through a therapeutic relationship rooted in empathy, unconditional positive regard and congruence. The therapist responds to the client as a unique individual at all times and adheres to the guiding principle that a basic, non-judgmental posture of respect, trust, honesty and care will establish an ideal relationship and environment wherein the client may achieve growth (Scovel and Gardstrom, 2002). The client-as-person, not procedures and techniques, drives the selections of music experiences and therapeutic processes (Garred, 2006; Ruud, 2010; Van Den Hurk and Smeijsters, 1991). Goals are ultimately understood in terms of their holistic, human value (Sorel, 2011) and often include musical terminology as integral to the goal itself. MT models that embody humanistic principles include the methods of Nordoff and Robbins (1997, 2007) and Helen Bonny (1998). (*Brian Abrams*)

humming

Sounding the voice with mouth closed with the intention of creating a soft, soothing melody or group harmony. Humming allows therapists or clients to warm up their voices, create a quiet sound and provide a nurturing effect. It also provides a closed-lip alternative for clients who are uncomfortable or reticent about singing. Humming is often used by *mts* for creating a calming environment. Examples include humming a lullaby to an infant or humming a melody to a client to facilitate relaxation. Humming may be supported by musical accompaniment. (*Robin Rio*)

hypothalamus

A primitive brain area just below the thalamus and above the brain stem that drives behaviours. It is important in regulating a number of metabolic processes. It secretes important hormones through the pituitary gland that regulate other endocrine organs in the body and controls the output of the autonomic nervous system. Its function includes regulation of body temperature, hunger, thirst, sleep–wake cycles and modulates emotional and affective behaviour. Music, emotions and food stimulate this part of the brain. Data by Menon and Levitin (2005) 'suggests that dynamic interactions between the nucleus accumbens, the ventral tegmental area and the hypothalamus may play an important role in regulating emotional responses to music' (p. 182). (*Robin Hsiung and Kevin Kirkland*)

improvisation as autobiography

All musical performances may be said to be autobiographical. This includes improvisation, which can reveal aspects – personality traits, musical history, life experience and frame of mind – of the improviser. In an MT learning environment, improvisation as autobiography may be used to facilitate reflection and growth. In this approach, parallels between autobiography as literary device and improvisation as life review are combined. Clients have opportunities to improvise their life stories, using instruments of their choice, while factoring in musical proficiency. The therapist and, if applicable, other group members, listen carefully to the improvisation, take notes and respond to what they have heard in the music. This feedback is processed by the client with a view to deeper self-understanding, self-perception and communication style with what was expressed. Rosen's (1998) work on autobiography offers analytical categories for autobiographical analysis applied to the analysis of an improvisation: representation, association, mood, experience, themes, events and episodes, colour, emotion, spontaneity, planned, aesthetic, authentic, identity, memory and meaning making. By framing improvisation through the lens of autobiography, an *mt* can listen for and perhaps ultimately standardize an assessment for the style and content of life expressed through play. (*Kevin Kirkland*)

improvisational styles

A set of musical idioms and conventions that can be identified with particular cultures; also refers to a composer's unique approach within a style of music. A style can contain several idioms, which are a set of defining musical characteristics or components working together. Styles do not exist in isolation; they often borrow elements or even evolve directly from one another. Each style, however, emphasizes particular musical elements or mannerisms more than others; thus, each style assumes its own unique and readily identifiable configuration. One major aspect of evoking a style is considering how the music is to be played. This includes following the rules of instrumentation, tempo, timbre, form, timing and other conventions. In MT, improvisational styles can skilfully used to meet client's needs. Some clients indicate a preferred musical style but therapists must often decide. It is important to fully assess clients' musical tendencies and offer music that will match their improvisational styles. Musical styles can be thought of as having personalities or characters and some may reflect a client's characteristics. Improvisational styles may provide a musical opening for clients to express their emotional and practical needs, thus addressing more accurately the aims and objectives of the therapeutic process (Lee and Houde, 2011). (*Colin Andrew Lee*)

improvised song stories

An MT verbal technique that encourages clients to develop the activity in their own direction by singing a song whose content is not preconceived (Oldfield, 2006a). It requires the therapist's ability to model the content and to adjust an improvised song story towards a therapeutic goal. The empathic approach to the client and their active participation in improvised song story supports the co-creation of the product which can be accompanied with either instruments or voices. The titles or issues explored within song stories may be specific feelings, ideas, images, fantasies, memories, events or situations. The song stories and the responses to them become personally significant in completing the client–therapist relationship by establishing verbal communication. They are used to reinforce vocabulary and to facilitate self-reflection, life review, and self-expression. (*Ivana Ilic*)

infant-directed singing

Refers to altered vocal characteristics of the adult when singing directly to infants and children, sharing many qualities of infant-directed speech (Trehub, Unyk and Trainor, 1993; O'Gorman, 2006). Qualities of the singing include a slower tempo, more energy in the lower frequencies, longer pauses between the sung lines, a higher pitch and vibrato (Trehub and Schellenberg, 1995). The key feature is a more intense level of emotional engagement characterized by a higher pitch level and slower tempo (Trainor, Austin and Desjardins, 2000), as well as effects on sustaining attention, modulating arousal and coordinating actions (Tan, Pfordresher and Harré, 2010). If the song is playful then the singing is more 'brilliant, clipped, and rhythmic', while lullabies are more 'airy, smooth and soothing' (Rock, Trainor and Addison, 1999: 527). (*Helen Shoemark*)

informed consent

Informed consent is a signed form given when a client agrees to therapeutic treatment for the purposes of gathering information with the future possibilities of presentations, publications, research, teaching, promotion and other forms of dissemination of the process or results of MT. It is important for the *mt* to explain both verbally and in simple, accessible wording the purposes of the consent and to articulate all the potential ways in which the material from sessions may be used so that the client can make an informed decision about how they want their information used and their privacy protected. Informed consent should not prevent access to MT if the client declines. Consent should be obtained before therapy begins and should allow for choice of what is being consented to, such as videotaping, videorecording, photographs, session material (intake, goals, objectives, outcomes, evaluation) and that consent may be revoked at any time during the therapeutic process. An *mt* should consult their association's code of ethics for more regarding their responsibilities around informed consent. (*Kevin Kirkland*)

inner rehearsal

Hearing a sung or spoken phrase in the mind prior to vocalization it is called inner rehearsal. Researchers (Norton *et al.*, 2009) believe that inner rehearsal may assist clients to recover speech using techniques, such as melodic intonation therapy for this purpose. The ability to rehearse an intended phrase prior to using intonation or its elements is a skill to assess for and encourage in clients with speech deficits, including stuttering. (*Kevin Kirkland*)

intake

The initial interview meeting during which a new client commits to engage the MT service. Intake consists of the client (or guardian) and the *mt* sharing information. For instance, the potential client will state reasons for seeking MT and summarize their diagnosis, health, issues, needs, treatment history and current status. The *mt* provides an overview of their particular service and the kinds of treatment experiences that will be offered. Together, they discuss realistic desired outcomes of therapy and methods that can be employed toward these goals. Intake appointments with a practitioner in private practice potentially include agreeing upon fees, length of treatment and signing a contract, and informed consent if session materials will be used for research, publication, presentation or other applications. It is possible that a formal client assessment will occur during the same appointment. (*Donna Chadwick*)

integrative–eclectic music therapy

A triangular (client/therapist/music relationship approached from several theoretical viewpoints (Rubin, 2001) that gives the therapist a wide range of musical choices for implementing activities and simultaneously requiring a clear understanding of the limits of targeted application of methods and techniques used. An integrative–eclectic approach allows the MT to be flexible in selecting methods and techniques and allows for creative and receptive MT use during a single session or over the course of therapy (Paipare, 2011). (*Mirdza Paipare*)

intensity profile

While 'contour' describes the shape of a melody, the way the notes rise and fall and 'intensity' understood as volume describes the loudness of a given sound source, the intensity profile is a qualitative interpretation of the felt intensity of a given composition or improvisation experienced by a sensitive and open listener. A rising melody is often experienced as more intense than a falling melody line but the opposite is also possible: two bars of silence can be experienced as even more intense than an *ff* coda of a symphony. Helen Bonny (1978/2002) developed what she called 'profiles of affective/energy dynamics' (2002: 312) illustrated by profiles of whole GIM programmes, while Trondalen (2002) and Bonde (2005) have developed, respectively, the intensity profile to describe the actual or potential experience of an improvisation or composition in an easy-to-grasp graphic form. Susan and Steve Rickman developed the software program, Mia (www.miamusicmap.com), to make a simple, easy to grasp intensity profile based on volume only. (*Lars Ole Bonde*)

interactive family music therapy

The term is used in MT by Oldfield (2006a, 2006b) to describe her work with children and families. Her approach is based on the premise that MT can support the parent–child relationship. During sessions with families, she used mostly live and improvised music, aiming to increase active engagement and motivate families to become increasingly involved in the treatment process. Other clinicians who engage families in sessions refer to their work as family-based or family-centred MT. They employ 'a therapeutic approach that encompasses the child in terms of the family system of which they are a part' (Pasiali, 2010: 11), providing a variety of both pre-planned and spontaneous/improvisational interventions. Therapeutic goals include strengthening family relationships, developing social and communication skills and increasing bonding (cf. Edwards, 2011; Nicholson *et al.,* 2008; Oldfield and Flower, 2008; Pasiali, 2010; Walworth, 2009). Moreover, clinicians may employ specific interventions that can contribute to the assessment of parenting skills (Jacobsen and Wigram, 2007). (*Varvara Pasiali*)

intermediary object

A musical or non-musical object linking client and therapist (Heal and Wigram, 1993). Ira Altshuler (1943) used the term 'intermediary object', which was later adopted by Benenzon (1997). Other scholars use similar terms. Winnicott (1974) uses the term 'transitional object'. Poet Karen Chase (2007) calls the object linking client and therapist 'the third thing'. The intermediary object is this third domain, ideally a symbolic or meaningful contact item, may serve as a bridge or pathway toward creating a sound relationship between client and therapist. (*Kevin Kirkland*)

intermediate area of experience

A term used by Winnicott (1971) to denote 'that area... allowed to the infant between primary creativity and objective perception based upon reality testing' (p. 13). The infant is afforded the illusion that the mother is entirely under the control of the infant. This illusion is held until weaning, when the infant discovers a transitional object whose role is partly to preserve the illusion of symbiosis with the mother (primary caregiver) to soothe the infant in times of distress or anxiety. In time, the transitional object connects to the world of objectivity (external reality). Both subjectivity and objectivity are connected by the intermediate area of experience, which can also be thought of as the psychic area of play, possibility and imagination. In later life, this intermediate area of experience incorporates the arts, religion, imagination and creativity in science. The space in which we find others with similar interests allows for the meeting of inner subjective reality and external reality. This area is where our lifelong struggles with reality testing occur. We then face the question, 'Did I create this or was it presented to me?'. (*Paul Nolan*)

inter-therapy

A supervised training process, also called 'inter-therap', that developed out of Mary Priestley (1994) and her colleagues' early work with analytical music therapy (AMT). Originally, the process involved three trainee therapists assuming rotating roles as therapist, client and supervisor. Today, the process more commonly involves a trainee dyad alternating roles as therapist and client under the AMT trainer's supervision (Scheiby and Pedersen, 1999; Scheiby, in press). Inter-therapy reflects traditional psychoanalytical training approaches that invite instructors and students to experience a session from different perspectives to explore ideas and techniques that may be therapeutically beneficial for clients. Inter-therapy can be viewed as a non-hierarchical form of MT for the psychological health of *mts.* (*Susan Hadley*)

intervention

A form of strategic action in which a therapist gets involved – intervenes – to facilitate the positive creation of change in a client. In an MT relationship, actions include verbal, non-verbal and musical strategies implemented by the therapist to evoke a response or desired change from a client. Verbal interventions include counselling or instructions to assist a client during musical activities. Examples of non-verbal interventions include the use of signs, symbols and gestures. Musical interventions consist of the use of musical activities (singing, song writing, instrument playing, listening, composing, improvising) as well as musical elements, such as rhythm, tonality, tempo, dynamics and timbre. In defining MT, Bruscia (1998b) said it is 'a systematic process of intervention wherein the therapist helps the client to achieve health, using musical experiences and the relationships that develop through them as dynamic forces of change' (p. 47). (*Shirley Khalil*)

intimacy techniques

One of eight categories of clinical improvisation techniques used by *mts* for improvisation (Bruscia, 1987a). Four specific intimacy techniques include: sharing an instrument, giving, bonding and performing soliloquies. These techniques are designed to promote client–therapist closeness to strengthen the therapeutic relationship. They should be used after the working relationship has been established when the client is able to accept greater therapeutic intimacy. (*Lillian Eyre*)

ISO principle

A term coined by American music therapist Ira Altshuler, meaning, "The music is chosen so as to be isomoodic (matching the mood) and isotempic (matching the tempo), to match and resonate with the "mental tempo" of the client (Farnsworth, 1958: 160). In many MT approaches, the presenting being, mood, and music of the client is matched by the therapist to bring awareness to the immediate state. This can build rapport at both nonverbal and verbal levels. The music and therapeutic process is then either maintained to continue an exploration of what is present, or change is sought in a therapeutic direction either guided by the therapist or that evolves co-creatively as energy is shifted and released. *(Kevin Kirkland)*

jazz music

A style of music first developed by African-Americans in the late nineteenth and early twentieth centuries (Southern, 1997). The style of music began as a fusion of ragtime, blues, syncopated dance music and brass band music (Southern, 1997). Some musical elements that separate jazz other styles of music are improvisation, swing rhythms, extended harmonies, syncopation and musical interaction (Sharp, Snyder and Hischke, 1998; Larson, 2002). When used in MT, improvising in a jazz chord pattern or idiom can provide a familiar framework and support for one's clients (Aigen, 2005c). (*Peter Meyer*)

Kenny, Carolyn B. (b. 1946)

Clinician, author, presenter, artist and educator, Carolyn Kenny has written and presented internationally on MT, indigenous studies and the role of the arts in everyday life, human interaction and social change. Her clinical and teaching experience spans over four decades, working in Canada and the United States and internationally. She was the founder of the first Master of Music Therapy programme through Open University in Vancouver, British Columbia, and also the co-founder, with Nancy McMaster, of the first MT programme in Canada at Capilano College (now Capilano University). She currently conducts a private music psychotherapy practice in Santa Barbara, California, in addition to being Professor of Human Development and Indigenous Studies at Antioch University. She is an Editor-In-Chief (with Cheryl Dileo and Brynjulf Stige) of the online journal, *Voices: A World Forum for Music Therapy*. Dr Kenny's book, *The field of play* (1989), an extension of her doctoral dissertation, presents a theoretical framework for MT based on the interplay of seven elements or fields that shape musical expression and relationship dynamics within each session: the aesthetic; the musical space; the field of play; ritual; particular state of consciousness; power; and creative process. Her theoretical ideas are expanded in *Music and life in the field of play: an anthology* (2006). (*Shirley Khalil*)

key

In tonal music, the key defines the set of notes that are to be expected in a piece of music, thus providing a framework for the melody and harmony. The key is determined and named by its tonic and mode (for example, 'A flat major' or 'G minor'). The tonic or tonal centre is perceived as the 'home' or 'resting' note in the key. The mode may be major or minor. All major keys employ the same pattern of intervals and pitch relationships; they use different notes only because the pattern starts from a different tonic. Melodies and harmonies constructed within any major key therefore follow similar rules and expectations and have similar moods and affects. The minor mode follows a different pattern, so melodies and harmonies in minor keys are similar to each other but noticeably different from those in major keys. (*Catherine Schmidt-Jones*)

language see speech/language

leadership

Showing others, modelling or exemplifying behaviour or way of being; taking initiative to proceed with a course of action, taking ownership for actions and/or offering guidance. Effective leadership in MT inspires others to engage with a task or challenge. Non-directive leadership uses therapeutic skills to help the client come to self-realized conclusions and learning. Directive leadership involves the leader providing concrete or specific directives and solutions to problems. Clients can also be empowered to take the leadership within an MT session for self-esteem and ego mastery purposes. (*Robin Rio*)

levels of practice

Bruscia (1998b) defined levels of practice according to 'breadth, depth, and significance of the therapeutic intervention and change accomplished through music and music therapy' (p. 162). At the auxiliary level, music is used functionally for non-therapeutic but related purposes and the service provider does not act in the capacity of a therapist. This work often provides the foundation for clinical work. At the augmentative level, music enhances the efforts of other treatment modalities and makes supportive contributions to the client's overall treatment plan. The client–therapist relationship is primarily musical or activity based and is not used as the main therapeutic agent. At the intensive level, the *mt* works in tandem with other clinicians as an equal partner or as the primary therapist. Music is used in a central, independent role to address priority goals in the client's treatment plan. At the primary level, MT has an indispensable or singular role in meeting the client's core therapeutic needs and issues, often resulting in fundamental, deep and pervasive change. Verbal therapy is likely to be an important dimension of the client–therapist relationship. (*Lillian Eyre*)

limbic system

A group of interconnected cortical and subcortical brain areas, including the limbic cortex, the hippocampus, the hypothalamus and the amygdala. The horseshoe-shaped limbic system processes emotions and basic drives. The hypothalamus controls the body's homeostasis, orchestrating sympathetic and parasympathetic nervous system responses. The hippocampus is involved in laying down new memories. The limbic cortex is a loop of cortex directly bordering the corpus callosum. The amygdala receives input from the hypothalamus, the sensory cortex, prefrontal cortex and hippocampus. The amygdala sends afferents to the prefrontal cortex and the hypothalamus, bringing emotions to consciousness and coordinating physiological responses to subjective emotional states. Evidence from lesions of the amygdala shows that it mostly processes aversive affective states, such as fear (Nolte, 2008). Some evidence from the literature suggests that passive pleasant or unpleasant music listening spontaneously engages limbic and paralimbic systems (Brown, Martinez and Parsons, 2004; Blood *et al.,* 1999); music can bypass higher cortical brain functions and directly access the limbic system where emotions are processed (Montello, 1999). Seated in the old mammalian brain, improvisation is a process originating in play in mammals. The limbic system emerged between 240 and 180 million years ago as the centre of emotions, parenting, social organization and play. And *play* is the device which not only permits all mammals to have fun but also gives them a means of mastering the skills needed for survival (Hall, 1992: 224). (*Charles Limb, Malinda McPherson, Kevin Kirkland*)

lining out

An MT technique where the therapist refrains from singing the final word(s) of a line or phrase in a song to encourage the client to fill in the missing word(s). The technique can also be used for melodic lines or rhythmic patterns. Lining out cues and supports clients in memory, vocalization and participation, similar to filling in the blanks. (*Naomi Bell*)

listening

Listening is a complex neuropsychological process. It is an integral part of the human communicative behaviour, which includes speaking and writing. Music listening involves internal and external auditory and neural apparatus (outer, middle and inner ear, specialized neurons, auditory nerve, etc.) cortical and subcortical brain areas (brain stem, auditory cortex, hippocampus, amygdala, limbic system, motor neurons, mirror neurons) and has significant effect on the body and mind. In music listening, numerous processes are involved (emotion, cognition, attention, perception, memory, body movement). In the listening process, we can consider six steps (Kline, 2002): 1) *hearing*: the physical response to sound waves or frequencies; 2) *attending*: selectivity, strength and sustainment of attention are necessary for effective listening; 3) *understanding*: when the receiver analyses and understands the symbolic or metaphoric meaning of the message in that interpersonal context; 4) *responding*: responses to music can involve body movement, emotion, cognitive appraisal, physiological changes, and so on; 5) *remembering*: based on short-term and long-term memory; 6) *evaluating,* when active listeners are engaged in intelligent processes to reflect on the several dimensions of musical works (structure, melodic contour, timbre, rhythm, timing structure, chord progression, etc.) (Kline, 1996). (*Gabriella Giordanella Perilli*)

listening attitude

Inge Nygaard Pedersen (1999) defines listening attitude as a core MT technique employing an ultra-empathic way of listening to the client's music and to oneself. Through deep listening, awareness can be gained about the client's feelings, intervention possibilities and timing possibilities. A listening attitude conveys respect to the client, and conveys that you are not distracted with other thoughts or upcoming plans, but that you are fully present and attentive. Listening, whether to music or language, may be a key building block towards rapport, empathy, and grounded presence. (*Kevin Kirkland*)

low-frequency sound therapy (LFST)

The application of sinusoidal sound in the 27–120 Hz range to the human body for therapeutic purposes, which also includes physioacoustic therapy and vibroacoustic therapy. Effects essentially result from two mechanisms: 1) physical, through muscular and cellular means; and 2) neurological, through sensory-based brainwave entrainment. Physically, sound vibration is sensed by tactile receptors in the outer skin (Merkel disks – vibratory strength), inner skin (Meisner corpuscles – vibratory frequency) and in deeper tissues (Pacini corpuscles – acceleration) (Johnsson, 2001). To avoid numbing these sensors, LFST is usually constantly varied in amplitude (power pulsation) and/or frequency (scanning). The physical effect is obtained at a cellular and lymphatic level, by increased fluid and cellular waste transport, increased cellular metabolism (Skille and Wigram, 1995; Lehikoinen, 1996) and increased blood circulation, as well as muscular relaxation from a resonance response. Within the brain, vibration hypothetically enhances flow of cerebrospinal fluid and speeds the removal of metabolic waste (Karkkainen and Mitsui, 2006). Although less explored and often undifferentiated in research, considerable health effects of LFST may result at the neurological level from brainwave entrainment, especially through prolonged application of a single frequency (e.g. 40 Hz). Contraindications include acute inflammatory conditions, pregnancy, pacemakers, hypotension and thrombosis. (*Lee Bartel*)

marking

Momentarily synchronizing with the music of the client(s). During musical play, the *mt* briefly synchronizes with the client's music to convey empathy and strengthen their inter-musical connection (Das, 2011). (*Kalani Das*)

mastery experiences

Kohut and Levarie (1950/1978) applied an ego psychology perspective to the concept of mastery as an ego function. A key premise is that early acoustic environments can present chaotic and disturbing sounds to the infant, with sounds later replaced by meaningful sound experiences. Dissonance can be used to arouse tension states similar to those in early childhood. Pleasure arises when tension is relieved through the release of energy summoned to neutralize psychological threat. When listening to symphonic music, for example, a large amount of acoustic stimuli may be experienced by the client as chaotic or disturbing, which initially cannot be understood. If flight is not possible or the need to withdraw is resisted then large amounts of energy are activated for possible defensive protection. To neutralize anxiety from the sonic assault, the client may employ defensive avoidant behaviours. However, tension is often created and released within music itself. When the client follows the reduction of music tensions, returning to a quieter dynamic level or, alternatively, rising to a climatic resolution of the musical elements, the client can abandon flight preparations resulting in a pleasurable release of the acquired energy. The ego has gained a playful mastery over the 'threat'. (*Paul Nolan*)

matching

A musical and non-musical empathic approach used with clients using similar rhythms, sounds, energy levels, emotions and body language. Matching is a key element to Altshuler's (1948) concept of the ISO principle where aspects of the client's music, mood, tone, body language, etc., are matched by the therapist. Wigram (2004: 83–84) regards it as one of the most valuable of all improvisational methods, a usual place to begin developing a musical therapeutic alliance, the building block of further exploration as found in the Sonata Allegro form. It is a validating method that conveys being heard. Related concepts include Bruscia's (1987c) use of reflecting whereas Pavlicevic (1997) speaks of partial mirroring to differentiate from note-for-note matching. Clarkson (2008: 155) drew upon Bruscia (1987c: 344), using supportive mirroring to reflect a certain element or feature within the client's music. (*Kevin Kirkland*)

material-oriented improvisation

A subcategory of analytical music therapy (Priestley and Eschen, 2002: 26) material-oriented improvisation is recommended for clients benefitting from structured improvisation (ordered–unordered–ordered, like an A-B-A format) where well-defined ordered material is used to anchor the experience of unordered play, which may represent a more challenging or new area of exploration before returning to the familiar structure, (A), once again. (*Kevin Kirkland*)

McMaster, Nancy (b. 1946)

Music therapist, educator and pianist, Nancy studied in England in the early 1970s, where she also trained in the Nordoff and Robbins method. She practiced MT with developmentally delayed children upon her return to Vancouver. With Carolyn Kenny, she co-founded the first Canadian MT training programme in 1976 at Capilano College (now Capilano University) in North Vancouver and has been a core faculty member since. She was coordinator of the programme for several years. Nancy is a regular CAMT conference presenter, performer and published author in the field. She has served for over ten years on the board of the Music Therapy Association of British Columbia and is an assistant trainer of GIM. Nancy has inspired hundreds of *mts* with her dedication and passion both for the field and for her students. (*Liz Moffitt*)

medical music psychotherapy

The application and practice of MT in a medical context, whereby the therapist incorporates aspects of the client's life world within the dynamic music relationship (Loewy, 2000). Symbolic association of instruments and cultural assignment of music, clinical improvisation, as well as use of transference and countertransference, are key aspects of this practice. (*Joanne Loewy*)

melodic intonation therapy

An approach developed by Sparks, Helm, and Albert (1973) to facilitate the production of language in clients with mild to moderate non-fluent aphasia following neurological damage to Broca's area sustained during brain trauma or a cerebral vascular accident. This technique has also been used to improve language abilities of children with language-delayed apraxia (Krauss and Galloway, 1982). The melodic intonation therapy protocol uses intoned phrases and sentences. These intoned phrases are based on three elements of spoken prosody: 1) the melodic line or variation of pitch in the spoken phrase; 2) the tempo and rhythm of the utterance; and 3) the points of stress in the phrase (Sparks and Deck, 1986). Baker (2000, 2011) modified the approach to treat the most severe cases of non-fluent aphasia by increasing the degree of musicality of the phrases being rehearsed by her clients. In this way, the phrases were more predictable than those stipulated by Sparks, Helm, and Albert (1973) and therefore more easily retrieved from memory; the musical phrases function as mnemonic aids. (*Felicity Baker*)

metaphor

Concepts of analogy, metaphor and narrative are central to a post-positivist discourse on MT and are informed by the fact that meaning in music is based on context-bound references founded in bodily and emotional experiences and transformed into words. Contemporary cognitive metaphor theory understands metaphor as a basic tool of cognition and maintains that, 'The essence of metaphor is understanding and experiencing one kind of thing in terms of another' (Lakoff and Johnson, 1980: 5). Many psychotherapists have studied metaphors in therapy (Siegelman, 1990), assigning special importance to the inherent tension and ambiguity of the metaphor, which enables significant moments of awareness and insight. The metaphor 'reveals and hides' (Meltzer, 1990) at the same time and its therapeutic potential is connected with its basis in the client's personal imagination and language. This type of understanding is closely related to the body and the development of body (image) schemata (Johnson, 2007). We use metaphors to structure our understanding of new knowledge within unfamiliar areas: based primarily on bodily experiences well-known concepts are correlated with unknown or little known experiences. Abstract and complex things are structured by something more simple and sensory. Two embodied elements of music – tension and motion – are fundamental metaphorical elements. Langer (in Noy, 1993: 127) maintained that, 'music sounds the way an emotion feels'. As 'a living form', music captures the form of human life and feeling. 'Music is a metaphorical image of actual life. Music analogically represents the principles of living form in a new "virtual" form' (Langer, 1942: 54). Thus, metaphor bridges mind and body, and the theory of metaphor transcends the classic dualism of emotion and cognition. Scholars who have applied cognitive metaphor and schema theory to MT are Aigen, Bonde and Jungaberle (Aigen, 2005b). (*Lars Ole Bonde*)

metaphorical music therapy

An individual method that combines the benefits of music with those of artistic and narrative creation. Based upon two words (metaphors) given by the *mt* at the session's beginning that link with the client's history, the client achieves a small musical induction metaphorical tale in the form of a collage and a short story. The procedure is performed as follows: 1) according to client's musical tastes, client chooses a sequence of MT called 'U-based' of 20–25 minutes duration; its effect, construction, and application are comparable to a relaxation session or hypno-analgesia; 2) as client is wearing headphones and listening to the music in a quiet room, client is asked to select and cut fragments of images in magazines; 3) at the end of the musical sequence, client performs a narrative and composite collage using all selected elements for about 20–30 minutes. The contribution of joint mediation allows the client to benefit from the effects of the 'U-based' method in a different context than the relaxation usually suggested and through therapeutic metaphor proposed and collage, to access to a creative non-verbal communication supported and stimulated by MT. Inspired by Munro's collages in palliative care and hypnosis techniques, this method by C. Jourt Pineau is used in France with clients whose pain was resistant to high doses of morphine that generated psychic withdrawal. *(Cécilia Jourt Pineau)*

methodology

A series of choices and practices about what information and data to gather, how to analyze it and other associated choices. Information gathered is based upon the research or inquiry question(s), although it may also be applied to the practice setting. Any terms (such as MT, improvisation, mood) need to be operationally defined; that is, definitions that help to describe the steps needed to collect information about terms and process used. Methodologies are described so that others can replicate the findings or adapt them, in the hope of making improvements or expanding practice areas. Methodology differs from method; the latter is a singular approach or technique, whereas methodology is usually a standardized, accepted or pre-established sequence in a therapeutic or research process. (*Kevin Kirkland*)

microanalysis

Microanalyses are research methods investigating microprocesses of MT (Wosch and Wigram, 2007). The subject and timeframe of microprocesses are changes within one therapy session or parts of it. Microanalysis is process research and based in quantitative and/or qualitative paradigms. One example is quantitative single case analyses. The three possible databases of microanalyses are video, music and text. All clinical applications of MT can be investigated. However, microanalysis is of special meaning for investigating smallest changes in clients and correlations of therapist and client behaviour, especially clients with special needs (such as developmental disorders or in neurological rehabilitation) or those with dementia. In MT education, microanalysis is used for systematic sensitization of students to the smallest details of client and therapist behaviour and experience. Applications of microanalysis have also been used as assessment and diagnostic tools for clinical practice. (*Thomas Wosch*)

mirror neurons

Highly specialized motor neurons discovered in 1995 by an Italian group led by Rizzolatti and Sinigaglia (2008). These neurons become activated in the same pattern whether performing or just observing a task. Mirror neurons demonstrate the neural activity that corresponds to empathy and the sharing of the emotions of others, as in intersubjectivity. In MT, mirror neurons can become activated in clients when the *mt* is observed performing an expressive movement while playing a musical instrument or singing. In clients with normally developed brains, the emotional character of the therapist's gesture is produced in the same area in the client's brain. (*Paul Nolan*)

mirroring

An improvisation technique that conveys empathy, often equated with imitating, copying and synchronizing. Bruscia (1998a) calls it synchronizing, meaning that the therapists' music simultaneously matches the client's actions. Das (2011) adds that this requires musical understanding, the use of visual cues and intuition. Another application of mirroring is as a vocal holding technique. Austin (2009) describes this as the repetition of a client's melody to provide support or to demonstrate acceptance. Wigram (2004) defines mirroring more broadly as 'doing exactly what the client is doing musically, expressively, and through body language at the same time as the client is doing it. The client will then see [their] own behaviour in the therapist's behaviour' (p. 82). The latter definition encompasses the activities therapy approach to mirroring found in Schulberg (1981), where mirroring is a movement technique performed in dyads where one acts as leader and the other as follower. To increase attention or extend range of motion, a hand-over-hand approach may be incorporated, although typically there is no physical contact as when observing your own movement in a mirror. The *mt* may lead, follow or provide music for two or more clients. (*Rebecca Engen*)

mixed-methods research (MMR)

A research methodology intentionally integrating qualitative and quantitative data analyzing procedures for answering the research question(s). MMR is defined with a coherent research terminology and is both a distinct research method and a philosophical worldview or paradigm (Cresswell and Clark, 2007; Tashakkori and Teddlie, 2010). MMR is a multiple method design distinguished from multimethod designs (more methods are used but within the same paradigm) and from an 'everything can go' approach where data sources, methods of analysis and concepts are mixed up. It is a basic pragmatic principle of MMR that the integration of quantitative and qualitative approaches is derived from the research questions with the combination of methods aimed at giving a better understanding of the research problems. Hanson *et al.* (2005) describe six primary types of designs: three sequential (explanatory, exploratory, transformative) and three concurrent (triangulation, nested, transformative). MT is a complex intervention and the need to both generalize results and understand phenomena and complex therapeutic interactive processes in real-world settings has created a tradition for combining quantitative and qualitative data which in the last decade increasingly is defined as MMR (Barry *et al.*, 2010; Bonde, 2013; Gilboa and Roginsky 2010; McFerran *et al.*, 2010; Pool and Odell-Miller 2011; Ridder and Aldridge 2005; Silverman 2010). (*Hanne Mette Ridder*)

model

Ian Barbour (1974) defines a model in scientific terms as a 'temporary psychological aid in the formation of a theory' (p. 39). A model can be tested as a theory through the method, the outcomes and an evaluation of all components from both quantitative and qualitative perspectives. The development, application and analysis of MT models may ultimately inform a unified theory of MT. (*Kevin Kirkland*)

modes of consciousness

First used in connection with *mt* by Bruscia (1995) to describe the therapist's experience of 'being there' for the client. Bruscia identified modes of consciousness or shifts in consciousness that occur when one uses the self as an instrument of perception to apprehend the client's experience. He described 'worlds of consciousness', which included the client's world, the therapist's personal world and the therapist's therapeutic world. Integrated with these worlds are 'levels of experiencing' which include sensory, affective, reflective and intuitive functions. (*Lillian Eyre*)

modulation

A change of the music's tonic pitch, such as moving from C major to F major. To make this change, one or more notes from the established scale will change, creating a different scale and promoting a different pitch as tonic. The definitions 'change of scale' or 'change of key' are imprecise, however, since a change from C major to C minor is technically not considered a modulation but a change of mode. Modulations between keys that differ in key signature by relatively few accidentals are often easier to achieve since fewer notes of the established scale are altered; these modulations are generally smoother and can often go unnoticed by the listener. Modulations by common tone are also smooth and can sound dramatic or spiritual. This is achieved through use of a common tone in the originating triad, such as C-E-G for C major, which allows for a modulation to a major key a minor or major third above or below the tonic. Thus, the note of a C major triad can pivot to A♭ major, A major, E♭ major or E major because C, E, or G can be found in the modulated key. The effect of modulating to a slightly lower key (e.g. the tonic a semitone lower) combined with slowing of tempo may promote relaxation. Modulating up by semitone can create energy and a more intense emotional connection to the lyrics. To make moving the tonic up by semitone smoother, even though the scales of these two keys will differ by many notes, one can use the tonic pitch of the first key as a common tone that is also found in the V7 of the new key. To move from C major to D♭ major, for example, use C major – A♭7 –D♭ major. (*Peter Martens and Kevin Kirkland*)

mood

A sustained, often pervasive, emotional state that is maintained over time (e.g. neutral, depressed, euphoric, anxious, or irritable) (Brown and Kozak, 1998; Andreasen and Black, 1995). It tends to colour one's appraisal of environment and self-representation. Information that is mood-congruent will be better memorized than mood-incongruent ones (Russo *et al.*, 2006). Music has been used for many years in MT for its potential to positively influence mood in a given direction (Särkämö *et al.,* 2008, 2010; Martin and Metha, 1997; Hendon and Bohon, 2007; Valentine and Evans, 2001). Scientific inquiry on the neurochemical effects of music is adding evidence for music's ability to regulate mood and arousal in order to better psychological and physical health indicators (Chanda and Levitin, 2013). (*Marianne Bargiel*)

motor cortex

An umbrella term used to describe three smaller areas of the brain responsible for movement: the primary motor cortex (M1), the pre-motor area (PMA) and the supplementary motor area (SMA). These areas are located directly in front of (anterior to) the central sulcus. Together, they control the body's motor output. The motor cortex of each hemisphere directs the motions of the contralateral side of the body. M1 contains a somatotopic map, whereby adjacent areas of the cortex control adjacent areas of the body. The PMA coordinates actions in response to external stimuli, including sound and music (Chen 2009). The SMA coordinates internally initiated actions. M1 has strong connections with both the SMA and the PMA and also receives input from the sensory cortex. The SMA receives most of its input from the prefrontal cortex. The prefrontal and sensory cortices both provide input to the PMA. The motor cortices of both hemispheres are connected to help coordinate bilateral movements (Fitzgerald, 2012). (*Charles Limb and Malinda McPherson*)

movement to music see **dance/movement**

multichord tuning method (MCT)

A non-traditional guitar technique in which guitars are tuned either to the I, IV, or V chord for the purpose of enabling certain clients to play the guitar (Cassity, 1977). Once guitars are tuned to the three open chords, a guitar ensemble may be formed by assigning each client to play, upon cue from the *mt*, a guitar tuned to a given chord. The original tuning, recommended for nylon-stringed guitars, was based in the key of E. Cassity further recommended that guitars with steel or steel-blend strings be tuned in the key of D to prevent string breakage. The original tunings were, for the I chord: an E-based tuning with the first string tuned to E^{1} (first E above middle C), second string to B^{-1} (first B below middle C), third string to $G\sharp^{-1}$, fourth string to E^{-1}, fifth string to B^{-2} and sixth string to E^{-2}' IV chord: first string tuned to E^{1} (first E above middle C), second string to $C\sharp^{1}$, third string to A^{-1} (first A below middle C), fourth string to E^{-1}, fifth string to A^{-2}, and sixth string to A^{-3}; V chord: first string tuned to $D\sharp^{1}$ (first D♯ above middle C), second string to B^{-1} (first B below middle C), third string to $F\sharp^{-1}$ fourth string to B^{-2}, fifth string to B^{-2} and sixth string to B^{-3}. The MCT method was successfully used with clients diagnosed with moderate cognitive impairment (Cassity, 1977). (*Michael Cassity*)

multicultural music therapy

Therapists may have to challenge and develop their own musical knowledge and abilities when working in multicultural settings. Culture-centred MT requires great awareness and knowledge of the role that music plays in both the personal life and culture of a client (Ruud, in Van Bruggen-Rufi and Vink, 2011; Stige, 2002a). If the *mt* knows the traditional songs of a given culture and the meaning of the lyrics, and is able to play them for the client, the client feels accepted and understood. Gerdner (2000) describes this need to individualize music for multicultural elderly clients with dementia, in which the music functions as a bridge between their past/inactive cultural practices and the present ones (Gerdner, in Van Bruggen-Rufi and Vink, 2011). (*Monique van Bruggen-Rufi*)

multidimensional music therapy

A term coined by *mt* Jeremie Tucker (2005), meaning the practice of overcoming client resistance and facilitating engagement by incorporating photos, objects, general knowledge and current events with music to reach clients of varied ages, backgrounds and interests, especially in a large group of mixed cognitive levels. (*Jeremie Tucker*)

multimodal psychiatric music therapy

A model of psychiatric MT for adults, adolescents and children based on the BASIC-ID model of therapy (behaviour, affect, sensations, imagery, cognition, interpersonal, drugs and biology) proposed by psychologist Arnold Lazarus (1981). Multimodal psychiatric music therapy is an individualized, data-based, accountability model that includes a comprehensive assessment of client strengths and problems targeted most frequently by *mts*. Client problems are referenced to music activities used most frequently by *mts* to target specific problems (Cassity and Cassity, 1994; 2006). The model provides additional materials, instructions and examples for treatment planning and evaluation. (*Michael Cassity*)

Munro-Porchet, Susan (b. 1938)

Canadian MT pioneer, Susan Munro-Porchet, MA, MTA, CMT, SFMT, was trained in MT at the Guildhall School of Music and Drama under British *mt* pioneer Juliette Alvin. While there, Susan observed a Nordoff and Robbins workshop. Their 'music child' (2005) concept remained central to her later work in palliative care. She then returned to Montreal and began MT at the Anbar Institute. In 1977 she was the first *mt* in the Palliative Care Service of the Royal Victoria Hospital, a service pioneered by Dr Balfour Mount, who made the inclusion of MT in terminal care possible. Susan's practice and publication of MT in palliative care has been foundational (Munro, 1984; Porchet-Munro, 1993; Shugar, 2009). Munro-Porchet was also instrumental in the CAMT's establishment, together with Bill Shugar, Darlene Berringer, Nancy McMaster, Carolyn Kenny, Fran Herman, Norma Sharpe, and others. In 1985, Susan moved to her native Switzerland, establishing the first MT programme in the Department of Oncology at the Kantonsspital, St Gallen. Susan contributed to the development of palliative care as *mt* and educator within interdisciplinary training programmes for healthcare professionals across the country. In 2005, she received the Swiss Cancer Medal and, in 2008, the Swiss Palliative Care Award. (*Kevin Kirkland*)

music

Music has been conventionally defined as the art of sound in time, or the temporal ordering of successive or combined sounds (vocal, instrumental, and/or mechanical) that express ideas and emotions in coherent and cohesive ways, via elements such as timbre, rhythm, melody, and harmony. There have also been a number of definitions of music developed and applied specifically within the field of MT. Bruscia (1998b), in the context of defining MT, defines music as 'the human institution in which individuals create meaning and beauty through sound, using the arts of composition, improvisation, performance and listening' (p. 104). A number of theorists in MT (see, for example, Aigen, 2005b; Stige, 2002a) have articulated and incorporated the idea of music as the aesthetic, experiential, social act of what is known as *musicing* (Elliott, 1995) or *musicking* (Small, 1998). Specifically in the context of MT, Abrams (2011) has suggested that music may be understood as a temporal-aesthetic, relational way of being-together, not restricted to the aural medium of physical sound. (*Brian Abrams*)

music acupuncture therapy (MAT)

MAT was developed in 1994 and is based on traditional Chinese medicine and modern science (Shushardzhan, 1994). In research, acoustic waves have been found to influence the conductivity of acupuncture points and changes in the activity of the vital signs. Musical-acoustic stimuli are transmitted through earphones placed directly on the skin over certain acupuncture points. Special musical-acoustic tracks used in MAT suggest healing effects and pain reduction (Shushardzhan, 2001). MAT can be used instead of traditional acupuncture, especially in cases of weakened clients or individuals who are afraid of pain sensations from needles. (*Sergey Shushardzhan*)

music as co-therapist

First appears in early literature on GIM where the music functions as 'co-therapist, generator of images, integrator of experiences, supportive structure for abreaction, entrance into the realm of higher consciousness, and facilitator of inner dialogue' (Bonny, 1998: 10). Music is able to initiate movement in the psyche, reveal realms of consciousness, evoke imagery and promote integration of mind, body, and spirit' (Bush *et al.*, 2002: 44). The term can be applied to a range of MT practices where music is central to the therapeutic process, honouring the valued role of music in MT practice. (*Sue Baines*)

music breathing

An adaptation of GIM that has been introduced by Swedish psychiatrist and GIM therapist Dag Körlin in the treatment of clients with complex trauma, dissociation and other stress-related disorders (Körlin, 2010). With these populations, regular GIM can lead to overly strong memories of trauma and alarm reactions. Music breathing provides tools for modulating these experiences to make them manageable. It involves a combination of meditative breathing integrated with music listening and imagery. Music breathing aims at the promotion of interaction between the parasympathetic and sympathetic systems, which is often dysregulated in people suffering from complex trauma. Continuous practice of the modulation of breathing – in the form of size, rate and space – gradually helps the client to self-regulate the intensity of trauma manifestations that occur on both psychological and physiological levels, including dissociations, anxiety, flashbacks, alarm reactions and affective experiences. The accompanying music is carefully selected to contain and expand the experience by generating imagery, thus facilitating grounding and mind–body integration. As opposed to traditional GIM, in music breathing, the client images in silence and the guiding and verbal processing occurs after the music listening part. Mandala drawings/paintings usually complement the therapeutic process (Körlin, 2007–08, 2010). (*Evangelia Papanikolaou*)

music child

A concept advanced by Robbins (2005), it is the fundamental belief of the work of Nordoff–Robbins music therapy. 'Music child' refers to the inborn musical self within every human, 'the source of energy and motivation that supports all developmental and therapeutic process in music therapy' (p. 30). It posits that musicality is innate in every child regardless of challenges, reflecting a universal sensitivity to music and its many elements (Robbins and Robbins, 1991a). Music child 'denotes a constellation of receptive, cognitive, expressive, and communicative capacities that can become central to the organization and development of the personality insofar as a child can be stimulated to use these capacities with significant self-commitment' (Nordoff and Robbins, 2007: 4). (*Jennifer Lin*)

music life plan (MLP)

A comprehensive music treatment planning and delivery system introduced by Chadwick and Wacks (2011). It is a sophisticated form of advance music directive, written when a person is healthy, to articulate wishes that may require implementation in the event of later incapacitation. Using an assessment named the MLP preference profile, the *mt* conducts an extensive music life review, during which the client is supported in evaluative reminiscence. The client determines music choices aimed toward optimal physical/emotional states of relaxation, energy, spiritual peace and ethnic identification. Then, the client designs a detailed treatment plan for uses of this music. It is communicated to the client's medical team, attorney and family. When a life change, such as a terminal or chronic diagnosis or other medical crisis occurs, the MLP is enacted according to strict protocol. Software specifically patented for the MLP serves as a delivery system for the client's music. This software enables clinical application in a variety of medical settings as well as nursing homes and hospice. (*Donna Chadwick*)

music psychodrama

During the 1970s, Joseph Moreno (1999, 2006) developed musical adaptations of psychodrama techniques for use in group MT. He exploited the possibilities inherent in clinical improvisation to implement techniques such as warm-up (musical and verbal), identification of a protagonist, musical role reversal, musical mirroring, and musical modelling in a psychodrama context for high-functioning clients. (*Lillian Eyre*)

music psychotherapy

'[T]he use of music experiences [active or receptive] to facilitate the interpersonal process of therapist and client as well as the therapeutic change process itself' (Bruscia, 1998e: 2). The use of music for this purpose varies according to the therapist's philosophy or approach (e.g. psychodynamic, humanistic, music-centred, transpersonal) and treatment goals deemed necessary by the therapist and/or client(s). Bruscia (1998a) outlined four levels of engagement used in music psychotherapy contexts, ranging from exclusively musical to exclusively verbal: 1) music as psychotherapy; 2) music-centred psychotherapy; 3) music in psychotherapy; and 4) verbal psychotherapy with music. Some well-known models of music psychotherapy include analytical music therapy (Priestley, 1994), GIM (Bonny, 2002), vocal psychotherapy (Austin, 2009) and group analytical MT (Ahonen-Eerikäinen, 2007). Music psychotherapy can occur in both group and individual treatment contexts. It is generally considered to be an advanced form of MT practice requiring specialized training and/or certification. (*Laurel Young*)

music therapist

An MT is a musician who has received training in the profession of MT (qv). Darnley-Smith and Patey (2003: 5) describe it as 'a vocation, involving a deep commitment to music and the desire to use it as a medium to help others'. As with other therapeutic professions, of paramount importance is the establishment of a relationship between client/s and therapist that permits growth and change. The *mt* will support their client's communications with approaches such as individualised improvisations or pre-composed music using a variety of instruments and/or voice. 'The growing relationship enables changes to occur, both in the condition of the client and in the form that the therapy takes' (Bunt and Hoskyns, 2002: 10). It should be noted that in some countries the title 'music therapist' is job-protected and can only be used by those with a qualification from an accredited training course. There are, equally, parts of the world where no such training is available. Consequently the term MT can encompass a wide variety of practitioners and practices. (*Liz Coombes*)

Music Therapists for Peace (MTP)

Edith Boxill's vision for Music Therapists for Peace came from expanding her philosophy of a continuum of awareness to a global vision. Boxill believed that *mts* can make a significant contribution to world peace using their unique skills (Boxill, 1988: 80), to maintain 'a conscious awareness of contributing to the healing of our wounded planet' (Boxill, 1997a: 1). MTP is described more as a movement than an organization, with no political or religion affiliations and adhering to the Universal Declaration of Human Rights (Vinader, 2008). Vinader writes, 'Music therapists have been extending their work outside the treatment room for more than a decade... in response to the trauma caused by war and by terrorist attacks . . . nowadays we are implementing our modality not only towards healing but also towards prevention, by supporting the creation of a culture of peace' (2008: 158). (*Sue Baines*)

music therapy

A number of professional MT organizations have developed and/or adopted definitions of MT. For example: 'The clinical and evidence-based use of music interventions to accomplish individualized goals within a therapeutic relationship by a credentialed professional who has completed an approved MT program . . . and . . . an established health profession in which music is used within a therapeutic relationship to address physical, emotional, cognitive, and social needs of individuals' (AMTA, 2011); 'The specialized use of music by a credentialed professional who develops individualized treatment and supportive interventions with people of all ages and ability levels to address their social, communication, emotional, physical, cognitive, sensory and spiritual needs' (Certification Board for Music Therapists, 2011); 'The skillful use of music and musical elements by an accredited music therapist to promote, maintain, and restore mental, physical, emotional, and spiritual health. Music has nonverbal, creative, structural, and emotional qualities; these are used in the therapeutic relationship to facilitate contact, interaction, self-awareness, learning, self-expression, communication, and personal development' (CAMT, 1994); 'The professional use of music and its elements as an intervention in medical, educational, and everyday environments with individuals, groups, families, or communities who seek to optimize their quality of life and improve their physical, social, communicative, emotional, intellectual, and spiritual health and wellbeing' (WFMT, 2011). Perhaps the most prominent definition provided by an individual is Bruscia's (1998b: 20) *working definition*: 'a systematic process of intervention wherein the therapist helps the client to promote health, using music experiences and the relationships that develop through them as dynamic forces of change'. Extending the aesthetic–social concept of *musicing/musicking* to MT, Aigen (2005a) has considered an understanding of MT as musicing in a clinical context, whereas Stige (2002a) has considered an understanding of the practice as *health musicking*. Based upon a concept of music as a *temporal-aesthetic-relational* phenomenon, and a concept of MT goals as intrinsically *musical*, Abrams (2011) has provided a working definition of music therapy as client and therapist working together musically to promote the client's musical health. *(Brian Abrams)*

music therapy assessment for emotionally disturbed children (MTA-ED)

Based on several years of both in-patient and out-patient psychiatric MT work conducted at New York Hospital, the MTA-ED (Goodman, 1989) is open-ended and outlines basic musical elements that the child may express. The interpretation of how, why and when the child musically communicates may be viewed in context of the child's pathology. Areas of description include: natural response choice, musical preference, musical responsiveness (rhythm, dynamics, articulation, tone quality, melodic line/phrasing, pulse, physical disposition of instrument, appropriateness of expressive quality), verbal associations, non-verbal reactions and client–therapist interaction. A final segment of the assessment format details discussion and recommendations for treatment. This tool was developed as a projective means of viewing musical response for the disturbed child (Goodman, 2007: 44–45; 59 ff). (*Karen Goodman*)

music therapy process

Depending on the methodology, the spectrum of the MT process can be detailed according to several interrelated categories based on the desired outcome(s): 1) educational; 2) interpersonal; 3) artistic; 4) creative; 5) scientific; 6) empathic; 7) redress; 8) connection; 9) expression; 10) communication; 11) interaction; 12) exploration; 13) influence; 14) motivation; and 15) validation (Dileo Maranto, 1993; Bruscia, 1998b). (*Kevin Kirkland*)

music therapy screening

An expeditious, specialized, non-standardized examination of a person for the purpose of determining their likely candidacy for MT services. Screening is performed when there are a large number of potential clients and time or staff ratios prohibit more desirable in-depth investigation through baseline-yielding formal MT assessments. Screening is accomplished individually, with the *mt* presenting live music and instruments, assessing responses in areas such as communication, social, emotional, physical/motor, cognitive, behavioural and spiritual domains. Significantly positive reaction to music stimuli in one or more of these domains generally indicates that the person is receptive and motivated, indicating potential benefit from MT. (*Donna Chadwick*)

musical audiobiography

This term is used by Bruscia (1998a) to describe the client's creation of a chronological music collection. The collection reflects significant life experiences that are given an audible narrative. The entire collection is then listened to in its entirety and shared with the *mt* either in one-to-one or in a group for various therapeutic purposes including disclosure, analysis and reflection. (*Kevin Kirkland*)

musical autobiography

A form of musical life review used to identify and compile musical selections and/or list significant musical events across one's lifespan. These selections and events are associated with important people, places and occasions; they express personal beliefs, feelings and values and are usually organized chronologically. This may help individuals to achieve personal insights, stimulate affective memories, contextualize past events, resolve difficult issues and/or connect clients to what is meaningful in their lives (Moreira *et al.,* 2009). Musical autobiography may also assist in bringing a sense of resolution to individuals and relationships in end-of-life contexts (Dileo and Loewy, 2005). Significant persons (family members or friends) and music experiences, such as listening, singing, playing instruments and song-writing, may be included as part of a musical autobiography. Bruscia (1998a) and Ruud (1997) were among the first to suggest musical autobiography as a necessary form of self-inquiry for both professional and student *mts*. It may also be argued that the act of producing music, especially improvisation, is itself autobiographical. (*Laurel Young*)

musical countertransference

A relational energy exchange occurring between therapist and client in the context of MT, which is four-fold. The phenomenon encompasses: 1) the *mt*'s unconscious musical reply to the client that is occurring in connection to the *mts* past relationship dynamics and can become conscious over time; 2) the therapist's unconscious musical reply to the client that occurs in connection to the client's past relationship dynamics; 3) a joining of both 1) and 2) occurring at the same time; and/or 4) an empathic musical response to a client's unconscious state associated with a strong identification to the client (Dillard, 2006). (*Lisa Templeton*)

musical development

A very broad topic that is initially considered from birth through adolescence (McPherson, 2006) and from varying cognitive developmental perspectives (Bamberger, 2006), with no consensus for a definition of musical development (Lamont, 2009). However, research concerning musical development tends to focus on aspects of musical understanding (including pitch, tonality, rhythm, metre, form, structure and style) as well as musical activity (including vocal, instrumental, composition and improvisation) (Lamont, 2009). Musical development may be considered as a process of enculturation and/or training (Sloboda, 1985). Early musical development details the musical behaviours that demonstrate auditory, vocal/tonal, rhythmical and cognitive skills seen in the developing child (Briggs, 1991); these have been contextualized psychologically (Briggs, 1991) and can provide a developmental framework when providing MT with the child who is developmentally delayed (Goodman, 2007: 86–97. (*Karen Goodman*)

musical encounter

A term used by Teresa Leite (2003) in the context of psychiatric MT, where 'there is more room for individuality and idiosyncrasy, while maintaining an interpersonal connection that is established between the participants at the level of actual sound features and even non-verbal symbolism' (p. 124). The term extends Frankl's view that the relationship between two persons seems to be the most significant aspect of the therapeutic process and may be termed as 'the encounter,' which he also called 'rapport' (Priestley and Eschen, 2002: 227). A musical encounter is similar to the therapeutic encounter or therapeutic alliance but, here, the music functions as an intermediary point of possible connection between therapist and client. (*Kevin Kirkland*)

musical form

Describes a musical structure that is created within a symbolizing process. Clear rhythmic and melodic themes may appear that can be further explored or varied. Musical figures can be characterized by phrasing and pauses. Features of the musical improvisation typically have a clear beginning and ending and these are prepared for mentally by client and *mt*. This is always an inter-subjective phenomenon between the two, who experience being equal to each other and feel free and autonomous to play, to think, to exist and to develop their own musical images and thoughts. There is an intertwining of the timbres of both players. During this process, the sounds that are generated in a musical improvisation are guided by something unknown (connects to the unconsciousness) to the subject. The music resonates with an inner awareness of something that is no longer experienced as external or unrelated. (*Jos De Backer*)

musical invariants

Global aspects of music such as 'structural constancies underlying surface change in local pattern features' (Dowling and Harwood, 1986: 160). These may include temporal organization, such as beat and tempo, as well as tonal regularities like key and instruments used in addition to stylistic consistencies such as the swing feel in jazz rhythms, the steady eighth note repetition of rock music background from the 1960s and altered chords used in jazz. Thematic invariants may apply to a specific piece of music while other invariants apply to an entire style. (*Paul Nolan*)

musical life review

The use of *mt*-facilitated active and/or receptive musical experiences by clients to evoke significant autobiographical memories for reflection, review and insight. This process often takes place in end-of-life care settings (Clements-Cortés, 2004) and can affirm for clients that their lives have had value and meaning. Musical life review can occur in individual and group contexts and may be contained within a single activity or may transpire over a period of time. Musical autobiography and musical audiobiography are two variations of musical life review. (*Laurel Young*)

musical mnemonics

The use of music as a memory tool to facilitate encoding, storage to long-term memory or retrieval of information from long-term memory (Gfeller, 2008). Music can be an effective mnemonic device for a number of reasons: increased attention, arousal and motivation associated with music engagement can promote sensory store and encoding, and can encourage persistence in information rehearsal. Rhythmic, melodic or rhyming patterns can assist in the organizing and sequencing of small pieces of information (chunking), which are then learned as a whole. Additionally, new information can be associated with already familiar musical patterns (associative learning) (Claussen and Thaut, 1997; Gfeller, 2008). These organizational processes, which help to facilitate long-term storage, can also be used during information retrieval. The efficacy of musical mnemonics has been documented with clients who have learning disabilities (Claussen and Thaut, 1997; Gfeller, 1983) and with those with neurological disorders and diseases (such as brain injuries or multiple sclerosis) (Thaut, Mertel and Leins, 2008; Thaut, Thaut and LaGasse, 2008). Musical mnemonic training, which is the use of musical exercises to address various memory encoding, decoding and recall functions, is one of the therapeutic music interventions used within neurological music therapy (Thaut, Thaut and LaGasse, 2008). (*Kate Gfeller*)

musical motor feedback

Uses music to stimulate the auditory cortex, helping to create controlled motor movements. This type of motor training is often used with clients who have suffered a stroke or other neurological trauma. Schauer and Mauritz (2003) believe that the recollection of melody and rhythm, together with proprioceptive feedback, leads to improved motor control. Musical motor feedback uses a sensory device, combined with a portable music player and headphones, to enhance the auditory feedback of the client's movements in a musical context. (*Melissa Telford*)

musical pragmatics

Even Ruud (1998) proposed a theoretical model of music's properties and potential to influence the body and mind described on four levels: 1) 'music as sound'; 2) as structure/syntax; 3) as semantics; and 4) as pragmatics, the last referring to the fact that musical meaning is always created through the specific interaction of persons within a given culture. 'Musicking' (Small, 1998) is a concept developed to describe the interactive nature of the musical experience and MT can be understood with Pierre Bourdieu as a social field, where 'habitus' and 'cultural capital' are created and negotiated (Ruud, 1998: 83). What this suggests is that *mts* must be aware of the potential conflicts in their field. '[T]hrough our music choices and our ways of being in our bodies, we communicate values that are not always in accordance with the life views of our clients' (Stige, 2002b). Musical pragmatics and the interpersonal nature of 'musicking' is a premise of community music therapy. (*Lars Ole Bonde*)

musical prosody

Prosody is the musical flow of speech (Wennerstrom, 2001). Musical prosody is described by Palmer and Hutchins (2006) as musical expression echoed in uses of speech. Common characteristics of musical prosody and speech prosody include phrasing, emotion, pitch, contour, non-verbal and verbal turn taking, emphasis, intention and meaning. Prosody may help to prime infants and learners to meaningfully understand a continuous acoustic stream of sound units. (*Kevin Kirkland*)

musical sedation

The use of live music entrained to a person's vital signs and employed with the intention of transitioning one from being awake to sleep. A model of music sedation was developed by Loewy (2009; Loewy *et al.*, 2005) and was tested against pharmacological sedation in infants from one month through to four years with efficacy in the level of sleep state achieved, the time asleep and efficiency in completing medical tests where sedation was necessary. (*Joanne Loewy*)

musical semantics

Ruud's (1998) theoretical model of music's properties and potential influence on mind and body is detailed on four levels: 1) 'music as sound'; 2) as structure/syntax; 3) as semantics; 4) as pragmatics. Music as semantics refers to layers of meaning relating to what is heard and understood as external or personal references of the musical signs or elements. Semantic meaning is always framed by and within personal and cultural contexts and, owing to the ambiguous character of the musical sign – which has *signifiant* (expression) but not *signifié* (specific content) – semantic meaning must always be negotiated between participants, who will never have exactly the same experience. 'We can regard all discussions about music as a way to make explicit value-laden negotiations between us and "them"' (Ruud, 1998: 80). Therapists often hear the music (experiences) of their clients as personal statements (metaphors or analogies) and develop a specific expertise in acknowledging and negotiating semantic meaning with them. (*Lars Ole Bonde*)

music supported therapy

Physical rehabilitation enhanced and supported through the use of music, based upon audio-sensory-motor circuitry interactions and the pleasure of engagement in music (Schneider, Schönle, Altenmüller & Münte, 2009; Rojo et al., 2011). Music mediated activities aid in motor training such as fine motor skills. Research supports that motor recovery through music may be linked to increased cognitive connectivity (Schneider, Münte, Rodriguez-Fornells, Sailer, & Altenmüller, 2010). Rehabilitation through music is proving to be more effective than rehabilitation without music-mediated approaches. *(Kevin Kirkland)*

musical symbiosis

Schiff and Schiff (1971) stated that symbiosis 'is experienced by both the mother and the child as a merging or sharing of their needs' (p. 71). When dysfunctional, symbiosis can refer to a pathological inability of a mother (or primary caregiver) and/or child to emotionally, even physically, separate. Mahler (1975) says that the development from symbiosis to individuation is of prime importance during the preverbal phase. Musical symbiosis can allow for the healthy merger of two individuals (therapist and client) followed by separation and closure. It was proposed that early musical (such as lullaby, cooing) and positive emotional experiences between a mother (primary caregiver) and baby set the stage for healthy holding and taking care of baby (Kohut and Levarie, 1950; Winnicott, 1971/1997). Diane Austin (1999, 2009) uses vocal holding to foster a symbiotic-like feeling and transference of merging safely as though with a stable mother (or primary caregiver). Shields and Robbins (1980) said that rhythm seems to 'enhance, embellish, and reinforce the underpinnings of a symbiosis' (pp. 239–240). Henk Smeijsters (1993) extends the concept to musical symbiosis where individuation involves active MT, a continuous process of merging and breaking up, of being together and being alone, and going toward one another and drifting apart: 'The nonverbal expression makes nonverbal solutions to problems possible' (p. 228). (*Kevin Kirkland*)

musical syntax

Ruud (1998) presents a theoretical model about music's properties and its potential to influence mind and body on four levels: as sound, as structure/syntax, as semantics and as pragmatics. Music as syntax refers to a specific level of meaning, relating to the aesthetic and stylistic rules or grammar of a specific musical style. We learn these rules or 'codes' as Ruud (1998) calls them, in both formal and informal ways, creating a competence of varying degree. A special competence is the vocabulary we may develop to formulate the aesthetic experiences into words. This vocabulary may vary from the technical discourse of musicologists to a layperson's discourse, which is often emotional and metaphorical. 'Our manner of talking about music makes visible how our discourse on music is embedded in a larger theoretical or ideological field' (Ruud, 1998: 79). The interplay of musical syntax and semantics is illustrated in an improvisation analysis by Ansdell (1996). (*Lars Ole Bonde*)

music-centred music therapy (MCMT)

Music-centred music therapy considers the quality and content of music as fundamental to an understanding of the therapeutic process (Aigen 2005a). To be music-centred is to acknowledge music as the primary therapeutic tool and to affirm that an understanding of musical structures (e.g. musicology) should be equal to those of non-musical structures (e.g. medicine). MCMT is not confined to one theoretical stance and can be adapted to all clinical approaches. The *mt* can therefore adapt a music-centred philosophy to such approaches as psychotherapy, community MT, behaviorism and GIM. (*Colin Andrew Lee*)

musicking

A term coined by Christopher Small (1998) designating the verb 'to music'. His definition: 'To music is to take part, in any capacity, in a musical performance, whether by performing, by listening, by rehearsing or practicing, by providing material for performance (composing), or by dancing' (Small, 1998: 9). Musicking is a social activity, not a thing. Musicking means music exists in performances, not in scores, everywhere where people gather to communicate. (*Hanna Hakomäki*)

musicmedicine

The use of music to assist in medical treatment, whereby music is used as the means of intervention or stimulus. The term was coined by Ralph Spintge (Spintge and Droh, 1987, 1993; Pratt and Spintge, 1995) and implies scientific evaluation of musical stimuli in medical settings through physiological, psychological and medical research, as well as therapeutic applications to complement traditional medical treatment. (*Joanne Loewy*)

musilanguage

A term popularized by musicologist Stephen Brown (2000), who has identified the overlapping evolutionary development of music and language. Brown theorizes that music and language were both communication systems that later split into separate, though interrelated, systems in human evolutionary history. (*Kevin Kirkland*)

narrative

The concepts of analogy, metaphor and narrative are core concepts in a post-positivist discourse on MT, based on the axiom that meaning in music is based on context-bound references founded in bodily and emotional experiences and transformed into words. Narration is a core feature of psychodynamic therapy and the meaning of therapy is in Ricoeur's (1978) words to define 'a more supportable narrative' of the client's life and problem than the narrative in which they are captured and from which they are suffering. Narratives can focus on specific problems or life 'scripts' or they can cover most of the client's life story. Universal narratives are found in myths and legends and they often follow specific structures or paths, e.g. the hero's myth. Metaphors are often brought together in narrative form, as narrative episodes or complete stories. Bonde

(2000) proposed three levels of metaphors in GIM clients' experiences in the music-listening phase of the session: 1) the basic level of the core metaphor, the discovery of hidden meaning through the imagery evoked and supported by the music; 2) the level of metaphors of the ego and the self, the discovery of the client's personal voice; and 3) the narrative level of joined metaphors, the discovery of plots and other configurations in the client's imagery and life story. Narrative is also one of three elements in the definition of communicative musicality (Malloch and Trevarthen, 2009), the other two being pulse and quality. (*Lars Ole Bonde*)

narrative inquiry and analysis

A therapeutic approach originated by White and Epston (1990) in which the client's life narrative is the primary therapeutic focus. Theoretical foundations include constructivist epistemology, feminism, hermeneutics, autobiography and postmodernism. Narrative inquiry is used in qualitative research, where information is gathered from clients' stories and storytelling. In MT, qualitative case studies provide information about clients in a narrative applicable to the process of narrative inquiry. Like hermeneutics, narrative inquiry is concerned with the analysis and interpretation of texts. In MT, a technique of therapeutic narrative analysis was developed by G. Aldridge (2005a, 2005b; Aldridge and Aldridge, 2008) as a way of understanding the meaning of what happens in the therapy process. (*Lillian Eyre*)

neurobiology of music

Both performing and listening to music activates large areas of the brain (Strickland, 2011). The transduction of sound waves into neuronal electrical potentials occurs in the cochlea of the inner ear. Action potentials are then sent from the cochlea to the auditory cortex by way of the auditory nerve, the brain stem and the mediate geniculate nucleus of the thalamus. The auditory cortex extracts information about the pitch, timbre, location and amplitude of the sound being heard, while the limbic system modulates affective responses to this sound. There is activation of the amygdala when listening to dissonant music, while nucleus accumbens (NAc), ventral tegmental area (VTA) and hypothalamus are active during perception of consonant music (Blood *et al.*, 1999; Peretz, 2006). The activation of the hypothalamus leads to changes in the autonomic nervous system, such as altered heart rate and respiratory rate. The VTA releases dopamine, a neurotransmitter crucial in the brain's reward pathway. It has been suggested that increased dopamine levels in the VTA and NAc is the ultimate source of the hedonic aspect of music (Menon and Levitin, 2005). Although both hemispheres are activated during the perception of music, it has been found that rhythmic (temporal) processing is lateralized to the left hemisphere, whereas pitch (spectral) processing is specialized to the right hemisphere (Zatorre and

Belin, 2001). During expressive performance of music, heart rate and sweat production increase but respiratory rate is decreased (Nakahara, 2009). (*Charles Limb and Malinda McPherson*)

neurological music therapy (NMT)

Thaut (2005) developed and defined evidence-based NMT as the therapeutic application of music to cognitive, sensory and motor function challenges arising from neurological disease of the human nervous system. Its treatment techniques are based on the scientific knowledge of music perception and production and their effects on non-musical brain and behaviour functions. Populations served include but are not limited to: stroke, traumatic brain injury, Parkinson's and Huntington's disease, cerebral palsy, Alzheimer's disease, autism and other neurological diseases and disorders affecting cognition, movement and communication (such as multiple sclerosis and muscular dystrophy). NMT consists of 19 standardized interventions (techniques), subdivided into three training domains: 1) sensorimotor; 2) speech and language; and 3) cognition; all adaptable to the client's functional needs and abilities. Treatment techniques in NMT are based on scientific research and use the transformational design model to standardize and apply the most beneficial music interventions. The transformational design model contains five steps: 1) diagnostic and functional assessment; 2) therapeutic goals and objectives; 3) functional and non-musical therapeutic exercises and stimuli; 4) translation from non-music exercises to therapeutic music exercises; 5) generalization of therapeutic learning to real-world application. (*Monique van Bruggen-Rufi*)

neuroplasticity

Defines the brain's potential to develop new neurons and/or new synapses in response to stimulation and learning. Until recently, it was generally believed that the adult brain (cortex) was structurally static; however, research now shows that the human brain is capable of self-modification and considerable reorganization following neurological trauma (Mateer and Kerns, 2000; Stein, 2000) and may have potential to regain and relearn lost functions. Studies with stroke clients suggest that focused music listening stimulates cognitive reorganization and enhances mood (Särkämö *et al.*, 2008, 2010). Neuroplasticity has also been considered to be the mechanism underpinning improvements in speech resulting from engagement in melodic intonation therapy (Baker, 2000; Baker and Uhlig, 2011). (*Felicity Baker*)

non-verbal

'Music therapy is an important treatment when one cannot appeal to well-functioning speech and thought' (Smeijsters, 1993: 225). Non-verbal (which can include paraverbal and pre-verbal) communication which, along with music, is a form of unspoken communication that may include facial expressions, gestures or body language. Non-verbal communication can be expressed through musical interplay between client and therapist, often bypassing or quietening the rational/analytical thinking areas of the brain. Clients may express themselves through their instrument selections, intensity and style of playing, symbolic sounds or patterns, silences and melodic choices, to name a few. (*Naomi Bell*)

Nordoff, Paul (1909–1977)

Co-founder (with Clive Robbins) of Creative MT or NRMT. Born in Philadelphia 4 June 1909, he studied at the Philadelphia Conservatory of Music and the Juilliard School, receiving honours and prizes both in performance and composition. He was Professor of Music at Bard College, NY (1949–1958). In the 1940s, Nordoff became interested in anthroposophy and lived at an anthroposophical community with his wife, Sabina, and their three children. In 1959, after a European tour, where he first encountered music's therapeutic potential, he resigned his academic career and dedicated the rest of his life to the empirical exploration of music as therapy. He began exploring music's therapeutic potential with children with disabilities at Sunfield, an anthroposophical special needs school in Worcestershire, England where Robbins was working as a teacher. Until the end of Nordoff's life, he and Robbins demonstrated their approach across Europe and the USA and undertook a series of projects. From 1967 onwards, Nordoff and Robbins taught extensively and wrote three books. Paul died on 18 January 1977 in Herdecke, Germany (Nordoff and Robbins, 1971, 1975, 1977). (*Giorgos Tsiris*)

Nordoff–Robbins music therapy (NRMT)

Also known as creative MT, NRMT is an improvisational approach to MT grounded in the belief that everyone, irrespective of disability or illness, can respond to music. It originates from the pioneering work of Paul Nordoff and Clive Robbins, who worked as therapist and co-therapist with children with special needs (1959–1976), initially within the context of anthroposophical establishments but then in a variety of settings across Europe and the USA. Nordoff's and Robbin's extensive clinical, research and teaching work led to the development of assessment and evaluation tools, as well as the publication of books (1971, 1975, 1977) and a series of children's songs, all of which formed the foundations of the approach. As a music-centred approach (Aigen, 2005a), NRMT uses music *as* therapy (rather than *in* therapy). The International Trust for NRMT was established in 1995 for the purpose of overseeing the use of the Nordoff–Robbins name and for maintaining and disseminating the original Nordoff–Robbins archives. To date, NRMT associations, centres and training programmes have been established worldwide and the approach is widely recognized and practised. (*Giorgos Tsiris*)

nucleus accumbens (NAc)

Consists of a group of neurons situated anterior to the putamen where it meets the head of the caudate nucleus. The NAc, together with the olfactory tubercle, forms the ventral striatum, which is considered as part of the basal ganglia. Inputs to the NAc include the prefrontal association cortex, amygdala and dopaminergic neurons from the ventral tegmental area and projects to the globus pallidus. Recent studies found that it is involved in pleasure and reward sensation, and mediates addiction, aggression, fear and the placebo effect (Salimpoor *et al.*, 2011; Kreutz and Lotze, 2007). It reacts to emotional music, perhaps through the release of the neurotransmitter, dopamine, which plays a major role in addiction. Similar to adrenaline, it affects brain processes that control movement, emotional response and ability to experience pleasure and pain (Gaidos, 2010: 27; Blood *et al.*, 1999). (*Robin Hsiung and Kevin Kirkland*)

objectives

The measurable desired functional outcome of an MT treatment intervention stated in specific terms leading toward a terminal goal. Objectives are concise and clearly identify what the *mt* is tracking with the method for data collection inherent in the objective. An example of an objective within the cognitive domain with the goal to improve decision making might be: given a verbal prompt, the client will verbally select one choice from a visual field of three during each weekly session for three consecutive sessions. (*Cynthia Colwell*)

open tuning

Used in both Western and non-Western music styles including blues, rock and folk. On the guitar, strings are tuned so a chord is achieved without fretting or pressing any strings. Open tuning can make use of open chords or other sonority combinations. In 'open A major' tuning, strings are tuned from the lowest to the highest string E-A-C♯-E-A-E. With an open tuning, other chords may be played by simply barring a fret with one finger or use of a slide. These tunings may facilitate unusual chordal combinations and interesting tonal clusters through use of drone and sustained strings. There are major and minor open tunings, even modal tunings, wherein strings are tuned to form a chord that is not definitively minor or major. Open tunings can make the guitar very accessible for those who have difficulty playing traditional chords and chord positions can be colour coded for identification (Michel and Pinson, 2005). This system of altered guitar tunings enables certain clients a success-oriented music experience for those who are unable to use traditional chordal fingering patterns (Cassity, 1977). (*Bill Ahessy and Michael Cassity*)

Orff music therapy

Based on the Orff Schulwerk approach, Orff MT was developed in clinical settings of social paediatrics in Germany by Gertrud Orff. She believed that clients would learn to interact with their environment through positive experiences playing and moving to music (Orff, 1980, 1989, 1994; Voight, 2003). Carl Orff's Schulwerk is a way to teach music based on things children like to do: sing, chant, move and keep a beat. The philosophy is to guide learning by hearing/making music first and reading/writing music second comparable to how we learn language. It is intended to involve participants in active, creative music making that develops the whole person while addressing social-emotional and cognitive stimulation (American Orff-Schulwerk Association, 2013). Gertrud Orff viewed four factors essential to adaptation of this Schulwerk to MT: 1) music defined as inclusive of word, sound and movement (elemental music); 2) structured and free improvisation; 3) a diverse instrumentarium; and 4) multisensory aspects of music (Voight, 2003). Several aspects of the Schulwerk naturally support MT: allow everyone to participate, begin where individual is developmentally, use multi-sensory approach, move from experiential to conceptual, design success-oriented experiences, use culturally specific material, view rhythm as foundation and focus on process rather than product (Bitcon, 2000; Colwell, 2005). (*Cynthia Colwell*)

ostinato

From the Italian, literally meaning obstinate. Refers to a musical part that repeats the same melodic, rhythm or harmonic sequence. This line is often in the bass and may be used as the basis for improvisation. In MT, this technique is commonly used in Orff Schulwerk (Orff, 1994) where repeated rhythms (such as borduns) and melodies are used to stimulate singing activities or to accompany a single melody or rhythm. Ostinatos are favoured in MT because they offer predictability as in improvisational situations together with potential feelings of release (Bruscia, 1987a: 247). Ostinatos are also used as an accompanying technique in clinical improvisation (Wigram, 2004: 165). (*Lillian Eyre*)

pacing

One of the 'techniques of empathy' identified in Bruscia's (1987a) work in which the *mt* matches the client's energy level in terms of intensity and tempo. (*Lillian Eyre*)

paradigm

'Is music a paradigm for wholeness?' asked the late Linda Keiser Mardis (d. 2011), a primary trainer of GIM (personal communication, 1993). This philosophical stance posits that certain kinds of music contain patterns conducive to wholeness;

that is, a therapeutic direction found within the music that offers the client pathways to a feeling or experience of completeness. A paradigm is a pattern, framework, concept or example, even an archetype. Through music's analogies, archetypes, representations, metaphors and structure, carefully selected or performed music can offer a container for an experience of wholeness, one that clients may never have experienced previously. Through the elements of music as well as qualities like texture, overtone, instrumentation, beauty, fullness, richness, sound, harmony and alchemy, Keiser Mardis proposed a potential philosophy, arguably a theory, of MT's effectiveness. (*Kevin Kirkland*).

paraverbal therapy (Heimlich model)

Developed by Evelyn Heimlich as a form of psychotherapy that uses non-verbal and verbal channels of communication (Heimlich and Mark, 1990). *Para* suggests that this therapy is used alongside other means of communication. Heimlich described paraverbal therapy as using 'various media as channels for communication in unorthodox, nontraditional ways. Separate components of music – rhythm, tempo, dynamics, as well as dance, mime, drama, and painting are combined for the expressive needs of the moment... Contributing to its therapeutic efficacy are the immediate connection of the various modalities with emotional experience and an anxiety-free, pleasureful atmosphere' (Heimlich, 1972: 65). She developed a series of manoeuvres using aspects of music, movement, art and others to work with children with communication, emotional, learning and other challenges (see Bruscia, 1987a). The skill of the paraverbal therapist is in utilizing the manoeuvres that are most appropriate for the child's needs at a particular time. Heimlich distinguished paraverbal therapy from MT, although both share many characteristics. It has been used with children in other settings, including hospitalized children (McDonnell, 1983) and a child who had been abused (Wheeler, 1987). Beyond its application with children, Grob (1981, 1998) used paraverbal therapy with clients of all chronological and mental ages and a variety of diagnoses. (*Barbara Wheeler*)

participant observation

A research method extending beyond naturalistic inquiry in which the researcher is immersed in the life of the culture they are studying to observe and understand it better from an insider's perspective, thus as both participant and observer. This allows the researcher to learn the values and assumptions of the culture under study by living and experiencing them (Jordenson, 1989). (*Julie Lytle*)

participation

The term 'participation' is sometimes used to refer to the act of entering a predefined activity and sometimes to the act of taking part in a whole, where you contribute and make a difference (some languages have different words for these two meanings). Used in the latter way, participation is a term that links individual and social aspects of human existence. In this perspective, participation is understood as a process of collaborative action and mutual recognition, which implies that individuals act together and create artefacts and/or activities that are valued in that particular community (Stige, 2006). Each musical situation is a possibility for creating a social space where there is room for different styles of self-presentation, including peripheral and silent forms of participation, as well as conventional forms, adventurous and eccentric forms (Stige, 2010). Participation within the session is usually seen in relation to possibilities for participation in society. An extension of the distinction made above (joining in versus making a difference) suggests that MT practices might prepare participants for adaptation, personal realization and/or civic engagement and citizen participation. If collaborative aspects are nurtured, connections between participation and resources such as social support and social capital can be established. (*Brynjulf Stige*)

participatory music therapy

Based on the premise of participatory medicine, the aim is a more trusting and mutually respectful environment where *mt* and client work collaboratively toward the client's optimum health (Carmichael, 2011/12). As clients continue to play a more significant role in guiding their own health care, clients who are educated about their condition – their goals – given the transparency of what the MT interventions seek to explore and uncover, are significant components of this approach. It represents a shift from therapist-as-hegemonic overlord (Garoian, 1999) where the *mt* is the all-knowing authority figure in the room who assumes to always know what is best for the client. (*Kevin Kirkland*)

pentatonic scale

This musical scale dates back to as early as 2000 BC. It is often referred to as the five-note scale because it comprises five different tones, within the octave, played in a specific sequence. The major pentatonic form is created, by leaving out the fourth and seventh scale degrees from any major scale. On the piano, this scale can also be produced by starting on F♯ and playing only the black keys. The minor pentatonic form is a natural minor scale with the second and sixth scale degrees omitted (1, flat 3, 4, 5, flat 7) (Wharram, 1969). Melodies based on the pentatonic scale are often heard in Asian and Scottish folk music, as well as in Celtic, jazz and gospel (spirituals) songs. These genres of world music are often known for openness, texture, energy and emotional depth. For these very reasons, *mts* will choose the pentatonic scale during musical improvisations. Additionally, the scale is considered to be naturally singable, is success oriented through the scale's lack of dissonance, and the overall pentatonic sound can add an element of novelty to a client's musical experience (Nordoff and Robbins, 2007). (*Andrea Cave*)

performance

From the end of the twentieth century, there has been a growing interest within various strands of music studies for the notion and practice of performance. The perspective taken is that music can be understood as action and interaction in social and cultural contexts. In other words, to relate to music is to take part in a musical performance (Small, 1998). Similarly, several MT theorists have described health as performance. Influential examples include the work of David Aldridge (1996) and Even Ruud (1998). In this perspective, health is viewed not just as freedom from serious injury and disease but also as a personal project and part of the individual's search for meaning in life. There are several theoretical routes that lead to a focus on performance in therapy and everyday life, with the sociocultural theory tradition pioneered by Vygotsky, the dramaturgical sociology of Goffman and theories of modernization and individualization as three prominent examples. In MT theory and practice, the relationship between musical performance and health as performance is of course crucial. Gary Ansdell (2010b) discusses processes and affordances of musical performance and argues for the value of working with clients across the full continuum of private to public MT. (*Brynjulf Stige*)

personhood

British gerontologist Thomas Kitwood (1937–1998) introduced the concept of personhood in the early 1980s at the University of Bradford in the UK. He believed that persons with dementia deserved the same status given to a human being by others in the context of relationship and social being (Kitwood, 1997a). Personhood calls upon the *mt* to view the person with dementia as whole, a composite of their physiology, personality, life circumstances, social history, and neurological impairment. 'Identity is maintained...largely on the basis of what others provide' (Kitwood, 1997b: 20). Kitwood opposed the institutionalizing attitudes of the day, preferring to personalize routines, schedules and ways of interacting. He advocated for empowering persons to continue to have independence, make choices and participate fully in their lives. Kitwood founded the Bradford Dementia Group in 1992 to develop best practices in teaching, education and research. In MT, personhood has been applied to a research study by Kirkland and Fortuna (2013) and Sherratt, Thornton, and Hattan (2004). (*Susan Summers*)

phenomenology

The study of the structure of experience. Philosophical phenomenology dates back to Edmund Husserl (1969), where experience is perceived as a phenomenon at which consciousness is directed (Mohanty and McKennan, 1989). In psychology, phenomenology is the study of intrinsic qualities of experience from the first-person perspective using, for instance, introspection, a method of the self-observation. In MT, phenomenological methods are integrated into the qualitative methods of questionnaire and interview. (*Jin Hyun Kim*)

physical rehabilitation

A process undertaken to restore a client's physical health, functioning and/or self-care abilities following surgery, illness or trauma. MT areas focused on rehabilitation may include coordination, strength, mobility, endurance, breathing, pain relief and training in daily activities (Thaut, 2008). Usually, clients find the act of rehabilitation to be both physically and emotionally draining. Music has the potential to act as a positive distractor and/or motivator while exercising. The rhythmic aspect of music can also be used to cue specific body movements and/or pacing. Therefore, MT has been used during physical rehabilitation programmes to encourage both participation and adherence (Clair and Memmott, 2008). (*Andrea Cave*)

physioacoustic method

An approach to low-frequency sound therapy developed by Petri Lehikoinen (1997). It uses low-frequency sinusoidal sound (27–113 Hz) featuring slow power pulsation to prevent muscle contraction, frequency scanning to treat muscles with a particular resonance frequency and, at times, directional movement of the sound. Lehikoinen developed the Next Wave chair system (Next Wave Ltd, Espoo, Finland) that was US Food and Drug Administration and British Standards Institution approved in the early 1990s for three claims related to physioacoustic therapy: increased circulation, decreased pain and increased mobility (http://www.nextwave.fi). (*Lee Bartel*)

physiological parameters

A quantitative research method applied both pre- and post-MT intervention to measure any changes in the physiological functioning of the body as a result of the intervention. For example, saliva sampling for measurement of immunoglobulin A (IgA, a measurement of immune function) and cortisol (a measurement of stress). (*Sarah Burns*)

pituitary gland

A small pea-sized structure protruding off the inferior surface of the hypothalamus that sits on an area of the skull base called the *sella turcica*. It is an important component of the endocrine system that regulate homeostasis – the stability of the internal environment inside the body of a living organism. It is divided into an anterior and a posterior portion. The anterior pituitary produces and secretes growth hormone, thyroid stimulating hormone, adrenocorticotropic hormone, beta-endorphin, prolactin, luteinizing hormone and follicle stimulating hormone. The posterior pituitary stores and secretes antidiuretic hormone (vasopressin) and oxytocin. MT is believed to activate the pituitary gland to release pain-relieving endorphins (Wong, Lopez-Nahas and Molassiotis, 2001). (*Robin Hsiung and Kevin Kirkland*)

play by number

The ordering of instruments or notes numbered with stickers or coloured dots. For those who cannot track traditional music notation, numbers 1 to 10 (fewer or more depending on the client's ability) placed on piano keys or similar instrument with a playable scale, such as a xylophone, that can be followed using the numbered sequence on a printed page, allowing for songs that fit within a small note range to be played. For example, *Love Me Tender* in C major would span the lower G to the F above middle C, or seven notes. Numbered from 1 to 7 from G (1) to F (7) allows the notes to be played by number while tracking a large print numbered score for the song that is laid out according to the flow of the verses: 1-4-3-4-5-2-5, 4-3-2-3-4. 1-4-3-4-5-2-5, 4-3-2-3-4. 6-6-6-6, 6-6-6, 6-5-4-5-6. 6-6-7-6-5-2-5, 4-3-6-5-4. Naturally, letter names of the keys could be used but, for some with cognitive challenges, the numbering system can be easier to read. (*Kevin Kirkland*)

playground

An interrelational space developed and co-constituted by client and *mt* that reflects primary caregiver–child interactions based on the concept of playground, a creative zone of playful interaction between the primary caregiver and infant (Winnicott, 1971/1997). Freud (1914/1957) first used the term in the context of transference, wherein symptoms could be given a new transference meaning through the child's sense of play. It is infused with spontaneous gestures and sounds that are heard and answered by the mother. In time, the mother or therapist-as-mother enters into play, resulting in the creation of a transitional playground, which serves as the basis of connection between client and *mt*. Cole and Taylor (2008) use gesture, movement, sound and music making to develop an MT playground for children and adults who have been deprived of healthy playground experience. Sanville (1999) said, 'For psychotherapy to work, both patient and analyst have to be able to play, and to play together' (p. 511). (*Kevin Kirkland*)

poetry

Often thought of as separate entities, poetry and music have a long historical connection. The root of the Greek word for melody, *melōidía*, signifies both poem and music, emphasizing their fundamental unity. Sung or intoned poems suggest a musical language, possibly connected to human being's original form of speech (Storr, 1992). Rhyme can enhance the intensity of a poem while freeform or stream-of-consciousness poetry may be used for a less structured and more success-oriented approach. Song lyrics can stand alone as poems. Used as an expressive and metaphoric language, poetry can reveal facets of the self while providing a framework for the memories, thoughts, ideas, symbols, images and sounds evoked (Fuhrman, 2002). Therapist, client-chosen or client-created poems can be used to express and reveal feelings and responses for discussion (Fox, 1997; Reiter, 2009; Jeppe, 2006; Masserman, 1986). (*Ali Zadeh Mohammadi*)

portraiture

A qualitative inquiry method that shares features of case study, narrative, phenomenological and ethnographic approaches. First described by Lawrence-Lightfoot and Hoffmann-Davis (1997), the aim of this method is 'to inform and inspire, to document and transform, to speak to the head and the heart' (p. 243) by capturing the 'complexities of human experiences with vigilance to empirical description and aesthetic expression' (p. 12). Stress is placed on the importance of the portraitists 'sketching' themselves into the portrait early on. Voice is central to portraiture. Voice refers to multiple ways of knowing as well as authorship and researcher's role, specifically voice as witness (discerning listener/observer), voice as interpretation (search for meaning), listening for voice (trusting that participants will reveal themselves in their own ways and time), voice in dialogue (eliciting participants' authentic voices through empathic regard), voice as preoccupation (underlying assumptions, personal experiences and theoretical perspectives that shape researcher's actions, observations and interpretations) and voice as autobiography (who we are determines the qualities of our interactions and the intensity of our questioning). To date, these *mts* have mentioned portraiture in their writings or research: Kenny (1999), Carroll (2007a, 2007b), Gardner (2008) and Merrill (2009). (*Debbie Carroll*)

prefrontal cortex (PFC)

Comprising the anterior region of the frontal lobe, the PFC is probably the neural centre that gives rise to human consciousness. The PFC processes all tasks involving attention, decision making and planning (Fuster, 2008). It is the neural centre of higher-level cognitive processes that require concentration on external stimuli and the creation of non-reflexive responses to those external stimuli. For example, the PFC is responsible for the formation of organized plans of action, language comprehension, language construction and working memory (the manipulation of internal representations). The PFC is also known as the frontal association cortex, as it simultaneously processes sensory input, emotions and memories. It may serve a critical role in altered states of consciousness, referred to as the 'hypofrontality hypothesis' (Dietrich, 2003). Of all the areas of the brain, the PFC has expanded the most, as primates have evolved, and is also the last area of the brain to fully develop as humans age. The PFC may react when a beat goes missing; during improvisation, a part of the PFC in monitoring performance shuts down, while parts involved in self-initiated thoughts activate (Gaidos, 2010: 27). The medial PFC region stores past memories and also serves as a hub that links familiar music and emotion (Janata, 2005; Fornazzari *et al.*, 2006). (*Charles Limb, Malinda McPherson and Kevin Kirkland*)

preventive intervention

Promotes the likelihood of the successful acquisition of developmental competence through intentional intervention across the lifespan (Hanson-Abromeit, Fisher and Merz, 2011). In a preventive intervention model, the trajectory of intervention is less clear than in a treatment model because intervention implementation occurs prior to an onset of a diagnosable disorder or disease (Zeanah and Zeanah, 2009). Assessment in a preventive model is based on needs rather than deficits. Needs assessment examines the characteristics of the client but also considers how individual characteristics are reflective of actions, beliefs, attitudes and behaviours of the cultural context (family, community and society). A needs assessment will also allow the *mt* to determine where a client falls on the continuum of risk factors and if a preventive intervention can be integrated into the context of the client's life (United States Department of Health and Human Services, 2010; McWhirter *et al.*, 2007). Preventive goals specify a desired difference between the current situation and the future. Objectives indicate proximal outcomes on a continuum of achievement and include a target date that is based on expected age of development when intervention is completed. Objectives should be measurable within a session and should be able to be tracked across time (Allen-Meares and Fraser, 2004; Collins and Dozois, 2008; Price and Lorion, 1989). (*Deanna Hanson-Abromeit, CharCarol Fisher, Beth Merz*)

Priestley, Mary (b. 1925)

Developer of Analytical Music Therapy (Priestley, 1975, 1994; Priestley and Eschen, 2002). Born in the UK, she was the child of famous English playwright and author, J. B. Priestley, and Jane Lewis (Bunt, 2004; Hadley, 2001). Her father was a vocalist with a strong ability to play by ear, while her mother was a trained pianist. Priestley studied piano, violin and composition in her youth, and trained and associated with some of the most famous musicians of her day. Priestley was diagnosed with bipolar disorder and, as a result, underwent psychiatric hospitalizations throughout her life (Hadley, 2001). She became interested in becoming an *mt* after hearing a lecture by *mt* Juliette Alvin. Through Priestley's work with her own Kleinian analyst, she became aware of psychodynamic constructs (transference, countertransference) which eventually shaped her theoretical orientation as an *mt* and provided groundwork for the development of her model. Priestley wrote *Music Therapy in Action* (1975), and began lecturing and training others in her approach (Hadley, 2001). She is currently retired and living in the UK. An archive of Priestley's published writings, together with those of others on the topic of analytical music therapy, has been compiled and made available at Temple University in Philadelphia. The archive includes all of her personal/clinical diaries and audiotapes of clinical work with approximately 75 clients, spanning the period 1971–90 (Bunt, 2004). (*Brian Abrams*)

process

Continuing engagement with clients through music in a progression towards optimum health. The process is a continuum of care and differs from process-oriented MT where insight and depth work is typical. Bruscia (1998b) considers process in MT as taking place over time, stating that process is 'a sequence of experiences leading to a desired state, rather than a single event that has an effect' (p. 33). Boxill (1986) defines process as 'an opening up and an eventual deepening of awareness' (p. 87). Rio (2002: 193) defined process as 'an organic evolution to an outcome rather than a carefully detailed and planned procedure. As a process, MT is not simply the sum of activities, but rather a flow between activity and reflection, movement and respite'. Rogers (1961) describes process as flowing, not fixed, and moving in a forward direction. (*Robin Rio*)

prosody

The rhythm, stress and intonation of speech. Prosody is influenced by emotion, phrasing, utterance and language spoken. Some authors differentiate between syntactic prosody (Brown, Martinez and Parsons, 2006), which applies to verbal speech and affective prosody, the emotional expression of spoken words and singing. Research is finding that music helps clients to perceive speech prosody and to decode emotions conveyed (Magne, Schön and Besson, 2006; Thompson, Schellenberg and Husain, 2003, 2004). According to Brown (2000), this overlapping of cues suggests that music and language have a common ancestor. (*Kevin Kirkland*)

protocol

The steps or components of an MT intervention, treatment, research experiment or assessment implemented because of its established or anticipated efficacy and based on pre-existing research and/or evidence-based practice. Examples in MT include Bittman *et al.*, (2005), Gold *et al.*, (2005), Harrison *et al.*, (2010), Erkkilä *et al.*, (2008) and Ridder, Wigram, and Ottesen (2009). (*Kevin Kirkland*)

psychiatric music therapy questionnaire (PMTQ)

A series of self-reported behavioural interview questionnaires used in the multimodal psychiatric MT assessment phase. Separate forms of the PMTQ are provided for adults, adolescents and children. The PMTQ for children is administered to a person significant to the child. The PMTQ manual cites reliability, validity and standardization data supporting clinical use of the PMTQ as a criterion-referenced test (Cassity and Cassity, 2006). Anderson and Krebaum (1998: 3) concluded from an exploratory study that the PMTQ appears to correlate with other psychometric instruments that assess symptoms and underlying personality constructs. Correlation coefficients are higher between similar constructs and lower for dissimilar constructs, supporting the concurrent and construct validity of the measure. The PMTQ, according to Anderson and Krebaum (1998), appears to be an effective assessment tool for MT if reliability and validity gain further support. Additional research is warranted to fully evaluate its psychometric properties. Strengths of the PMTQ are that it: 1) provides useful clinical information for treatment planning; 2) is easily administered and acceptable in clinical practice; and 3) may withstand the rigorous review of third-party funding providers or sponsors who make decisions about funding treatment. The PMTQ is recommended as one appropriate option for MT assessment in psychiatric settings. It appears to provide clinically useful data that may be used to evaluate progress during the course of treatment. (*Michael Cassity*)

psychoanalytical music therapy

A form of music-centred psychotherapy, a client–therapist exchange through musical improvisation or music listening. It aims to make possible an analytical therapeutic process. The psychoanalytical therapeutic frame is based on theories of Freud (1975), Winnicott (1960a, 1960b), Klein (1961/1984), Bion (Lipgar and Pines, 2003) and others. Interventions include use of transference, countertransference, holding, containment, projective identification and free-floating attention. Other MT phenomena include therapeutic provocation, anticipating inner silence, musical reverie and post-resonation (De Backer, 2008), with the aim to reduce or eliminate psychic suffering, conflicts, disorders and related complaints. Clients unable to actively participate in improvisation (because of strong defences, aphasia, dementia, motor restrictions, etc.) can find the musical improvisation present based on their affective resonance. This stance both widens and provides evidence for the unique significance of MT for psychological health needs traditional psychotherapy cannot address. Psychic problems are given shape in musical form. On this musical-symbolic level, the process of musical improvisation or music listening occurs in tandem with verbal reflection. This offers the possibility of conscious or unconscious layers of the psyche to tap often untapped frontiers seen as a prerequisite for positive therapeutic development. (*Jos De Backer*)

psychodynamic music therapy

An approach to MT that is founded on certain principles and theories of psychoanalysis, such as transference, countertransference, the unconscious and the mechanisms of defence. The therapeutic process is based on the relationship that is formed between the *mt* and the client and the attribution of conscious and unconscious meaning to everything that is unravelled during the sessions. Improvised music, created by both client and *mt*, is the facilitating medium. MT interest in psychoanalytical concepts began in the last quarter of the twentieth century (see, for example, Alvin, 1975; Priestley, 1975; Steele, 1984; Bruscia,

1987b; De Backer, 1993) but has been greatly expanding during the last two decades. Bruscia (1989b) placed PMT as a branch of music psychotherapy. Fundamental concepts that have been incorporated in this approach include also Freudian and post-Freudian theories of the mind, Klein's two mental positions, the theory of object relations, of self-psychology, Winnicott's holding and transitional objects, Bion's (1962, 1970) containment and basic assumptions and Foulkes' (1973/1990) group matrix. In the development and analysis of MT techniques, PMT has also been informed by the natural evolution of the mother–infant relationship and interaction (Stern, 1977). Techniques analyzed in this way include contextualization, reflection and variation (Woodcock, 1987). Shields and Robbins (1980) also present a psychodynamic theory of music (*Anthi Agrotou*)

psychodynamic voice therapy

Psychodynamic approaches stem from Freud's psychoanalytical approach and include those theories in psychology that see human functioning as based on the interaction of unconscious and conscious forces within. A psychodynamic application to voice therapy uses breath, sound, vocal improvisation, song and dialogue to facilitate intra-psychic and interpersonal growth and change. Vocal psychotherapy sessions may include the techniques of vocal holding, free associative singing, vocal improvisation and toning (Austin, 2009). (*Melissa Telford*)

psychological entrainment

Entrainment or 'phase locking' is literally getting on the same wavelength, which metaphorically refers to what can be described as psychological entrainment – two individuals or an individual and a group arriving at a consonance and acceptance manifest through qualities such as agreement of ideas, matched energy levels or rate of talking. A leader may first match a group's energy level and then take them to a new level, often referred to as 'pumping up an audience'. Specific interpersonal and emotional intelligence competencies are involved as well as communication strategies. Recent research points to gamma brainwave activity (30–100 Hz) involved in the selection and attention process required for psychological entrainment (Colgin *et al.,* 2009). (*Lee Bartel*)

psychosocial rehabilitation model of music therapy

One of the components of comprehensive community-based mental health care, also called the clubhouse model. The premise is that a person with a mental illness is more than the sum of their illness and can be rehabilitated back into society and can make a recovery to their optimum ability. It enables clients to acquire or regain the practical skills needed to live and socialize in the community and teaches them how to cope with their challenges (World Health Organization, 2001). MT emphasizes the here-and-now immediacy of processing, development of social skills, leisure activities, group cohesion, personal worth, right and responsibility for self-determination and focuses on strengths rather than pathologies and aims to reduce stigmas associated with mental illness (Chhina, 2004). By extension, this model can also be used in MT to address eye contact, sitting posture, hand and foot movements and other targeted behaviours (Krakouer *et al.*, 2001). (*Kevin Kirkland*)

psychotherapy-oriented music therapy

This approach can be rooted in several methods such as the Bonny Method of GIM, process-oriented improvisation methods including Priestley's (1975, 1994; Priestley and Eschen, 2002) analytical music therapy and diverse interventions such as song writing, lyric analysis, vocal methods (Austin, 1999, 2009; Newham, 1999) and creative arts experiences. Psychotherapy can occur on both non-verbal and verbal levels and across a range of populations (Dileo Maranto, 1993: 96). Historically, psychotherapeutic approaches with children have focused primarily on creative play without insight-oriented verbal processing, though play can be effective for persons of any age. (*Kevin Kirkland*)

qualitative research

Refers to scientific enquiries emanating from qualitative data (text, narratives, arts) distinguished from quantitative research (based on quantitative/numerical data). The focus of the research problem/questions is the exploration or description of interactions, events, cultures, processes, understandings, experiences or the meaning of certain phenomena. As a consequence, the collection of data may include the use of narratives, interviews, observations, artefacts, documents, focus group discussions and audio-video material. The nature of qualitative research is inductive (versus hypothetico-deductive) with theory evolving from data; ideographic (versus nomotetic) as data are seen as particular and unique; and constructivistic (versus positivistic) as meaning is constructed by the researcher engaged in the field. In MT research, the rationale for choosing qualitative methods is the wish to explore the therapists' 'experiences with patients and clients' (Wheeler and Kenny, 2005: 60) and the 'interest in generating clinically relevant research findings (Aigen, 2008: 258)'. Three primary methods used in qualitative MT research are grounded theory, naturalistic inquiry and phenomenology (Aigen, 2008). The complexity of qualitative MT research calls for comprehensive evaluation models such as the integral model (Abrams, 2005) and EPICURE (Stige, Malterud and Midtgarden, 2009). (*Hanne Mette Ridder and Orii McDermott*)

qualitative research credibility

Usually determined by trustworthiness of the findings. However, assessing the quality of qualitative research is complex, owing to the diversity of ontological, epistemological and methodological approaches (Spencer *et al.*, 2003; Stige, 2002c). Lincoln and Guba (1985, 1986) proposed the criteria of trustworthiness as: credibility (internal validity), transferability (external validity), dependability (reliability) and confirmability (objectivity). Various checklists, guidelines and assessment tools for quality assessment of qualitative research have been developed (see, for example, Malterud 2001a, 2001b; Mays and Pope, 1995; Tong, Sainsbury and Craig, 2007). Others argued that the use of checklists is not applicable to qualitative research and leads to technical essentialism (Barbour 2001; 2003). Bruscia (1998d) reviewed MT literature to identify the ideas of quality expressed in qualitative research writing and listed 16 items, including musical integrity and artistry. Stige *et al.* (2009c) proposed criteria for evaluation of qualitative research using the acronym EPICURE: engagement, processing, interpretation, critique, usefulness, relevance and ethics. Despite diverse views on qualitative research credibility, there is an understanding that rigor of qualitative research is achieved by ethical conduct, reflexivity, attention to negative cases and transferability (Creswell and Miller, 2000; Mays and Pope, 2000; Patton, 1999; Spencer *et al.*, 2003, Wheeler and Kenny, 2005). (*Orii McDermott and Hanne Mette Ridder*)

race

Prior to the fifteenth century, race was based on common descent, such as nation and tribe. As such, there were large numbers of human groupings. In the sixteenth and seventeenth centuries, European scientists hypothesized physical, social and cultural differences between human groups but rarely used the term 'race'. During the eighteenth century, European scientists defined race as a biological concept and associated it with biological and psychological traits, innate and unchangeable, often accompanied by demeaning implications. Blumenbach (1779) divided the human species into five subcategories distinguished by skin colour and other phenotypic markers: Caucasian (White), Mongolian (Yellow), Malayan (Brown), Ethiopian (later Negro) (Black) and American (Red). Other scientists of the period supported the classification of race as a valid scientific category and used it to predict and explain individual and group behaviour and to account for alleged differences in moral character and intelligence. In the twentieth century, Huxley and Haddon (1936) challenged scientific concepts that suggested the superiority and inferiority of certain races but held to the view that there were significant social differences between racial groups. In the mid-twentieth century, social scientists described race not as a biological objective reality but as a social construct or lived reality that some people use to talk about themselves and others. (*Susan Hadley*)

randomized controlled trial (RCT)

Heralded as the gold standard for assessing the effectiveness of an intervention. It consists of participants/subjects assigned at random to a treatment group and to a control group that does not receive the intervention, receives an alternate intervention or receives the treatment after the control group (Jadad and Enkin, 2007: 1–10). Treatment effects are monitored and recorded for both groups using standardized tests, scans and other measurement instruments. In MT, the intervention involves testing a protocol that can be applied consistently either very strictly or with inclusion of the client's needs and abilities as a necessary variable and component (Smeijsters, 2006). (*Kevin Kirkland*)

rap as therapy

Rap has been used in therapy since the 1980s by *mts*, psychologists, social workers and poetry therapists (Elligan, 2004). Listening to rap can trigger a profound response that stimulates powerful and insightful discussions around personal narratives, stories filled with pain, loss, grief and joy. Performing rap and modifying it allows for a greater sense of ownership of the music, providing the client with a sense of pride and positive personal creative expression and it functions as a vehicle for clients to perform their identities. Creating original raps allows clients to incorporate their identities and to rap about an array of experiences that are intra-psychologically and socially relevant to them. Improvising (freestyling) rap prepares clients to be able to deal effectively with unexpected and challenging situations, stressing how decisions made on the spot can lead to potentially life-changing consequences for which they must be learn to accept responsibility. Rap therapy not only facilitates the expression of manifest and latent content but also invites individuals to find their voice; in many cases, something they may have been denied. (*Susan Hadley*)

rapport

Viktor Frankl (2004) said that the therapeutic relationship (therapeutic alliance) between client and therapist supersedes the importance of method or technique for effective therapy and is based on the development of rapport with the client through safety, trust and meaningful connection (Eschen, 2002: 227). Rapport is a characteristic of interaction where *mt* and client are 'on the same wavelength'. Rapport can also be built through verbally and non-verbally matching or reflecting emotions, affect, body language, empathy, eye contact, respect, attentive/active listening, breathing, musically rendering the client's mood and a range of improvisation techniques that foster a sense of being heard and understood. Rapport can be influenced by the way the *mt* behaves, looks and sounds, by skills acquired (such as asking a perceptive question), ethics, beliefs and values, purpose in life and the capacity to be genuine and authentic where appropriate. (*Kevin Kirkland*)

receptive music therapy (RMT)

A generic term for MT models that use music listening applications in clinical practice. In receptive music therapy, the *mt* administers pre-recorded or live music to the client, who, in turn, is the recipient of the music experience, as distinct from being an active music maker (Grocke and Wigram, 2007b; Wigram, Pedersen and Bonde, 2002a). There are various styles of music used during receptive music therapy experiences, selected or designed according to the therapeutic aims and purposes, with a focus on physical, emotional, intellectual, aesthetic or spiritual aspects of the music (Bruscia, 1998e). The most internationally renowned model of receptive music therapy is GIM (Wigram, Pedersen and Bonde, 2002a) but there are several models and procedures worldwide, amongst them Schwabe's regulative music therapy, models for music relaxation, somatic-based experiences, such as vibroacoustic therapy, music-appreciation activities, song reminiscence techniques, and many others (Grocke and Wigram, 2007). (*Evangelia Papanikolaou*)

reconstructive music therapy

Wheeler (1983) classified levels of music psychotherapy based on Wolberg's (1977) psychotherapeutic levels. At the reconstructive level, the *mt* uses music to evoke unconscious or repressed feelings, images or conflicts that are processed through music and verbal discussion. The goal is to re-experience and work through past situations that were not adequately resolved, thereby promoting insight that will lead to change through a reorganization of the personality. (*Lillian Eyre*)

recovery model of music therapy

Ronald Borczon (1997) created a six-step MT recovery process for clients dealing with issues of substance abuse, dependency, co-dependence and depression (p. 117). The six steps are: 1) survival; 2) awakening of emergent awareness; 3) core issues; 4) transformations; 5) integration; 6) genesis (spirituality). The pathway deals with survivorship, working through triggers, dealing with distorted beliefs, making changes of thoughts, behaviours and actions, letting go, integrating parts and engaging in renewal and, finally, regenerating, finding meaning through spiritual experiences and being creative and harmonious. (*Kevin Kirkland*)

redirection techniques

Bruscia (1987c) used the term as one of eight categories of clinical improvisation techniques used by an *mt* in improvisation procedures. Eight specific redirection techniques were defined in this context: introducing change, differentiating, modulating, intensifying, calming, intervening, reacting and analogizing. (*Lillian Eyre*)

reductionism

A philosophical stance that posits that the whole can be explained in terms of the parts, which is the opposite of 'holism' where the unique properties of the parts cannot paint a full representation of the whole. This is the challenge when researching the effects of MT, where it is often impossible to separate out what it is within the music that has a positive effect; i.e. the rhythm, melody, pitches, tonality, associations, instrumentation, etc. (Kohl, 1992). (*Kevin Kirkland*)

re-educative music therapy

Wheeler (1983) classified levels of music psychotherapy based on Wolberg (1977). At the re-educative level, the *mt* uses music intensively in a supportive treatment to help the client to learn new ways of solving problems. The music itself is an indispensable aspect of therapy, as it is used to elicit cognitive and emotional reactions that are discussed, to evoke greater insight and improved functioning for the client. (*Lillian Eyre*)

referential techniques

Used in connection with clinical improvisation by Bruscia (1987c, 1998a), it refers to improvisations that use an instrument or voice to portray (represent) a non-musical concept in sound. This concept could be a feeling, idea, title, image, person, event or experience. Referential techniques are one of eight categories of improvisational techniques and specifically include the following seven techniques: pairing, symbolizing, recollecting, free-associating, projecting, fantasizing and storytelling. (*Lillian Eyre*)

reflexivity

The ability to think of oneself in relation to others is often called reflexivity. It involves moving between a first-person and third-person perspective and it evolves in dialogue. Consequently, it also includes the second-person perspective. In MT, reflexivity in and through musical activity is crucial, in ways that could be compared to the way in which rituals provide occasions for a community to view itself critically (Stige, 2002a). Social theorists argue that reflexivity is increasingly important in modern societies, where identity is a personal project rather than an inherent status (Beck, Giddens and Lash, 1994). Reflexivity has also become increasingly important in the discussion of qualitative research, where the process of articulating and evaluating questions underlying a study is prominent (Finlay and Gough, 2003). Reflexivity, then, illuminates the relationships between the knower and the objects and processes studied. In this perspective, what is known is influenced by the circumstances in which this is known, including the subject position of the researcher. A reflexive methodology (Alvesson and Sköldberg, 2009) takes these processes into consideration and goes beyond the investigator's scrutiny of personal context and pre-understanding to include scrutiny of research design and techniques and the interpretive, critical and rhetorical aspects of the research process. (*Brynjulf Stige*)

reflex-resonant theory of music therapy

Multilevel mechanisms of music influence the human organism (Shushardzhan, Shushardzhan and Eremina, 2008). This theory proposes that musical sounds within the range of hearing 20–20,000 Hz are always accompanied by infrasonic fluctuations (Novytskaya, 2009) that together have complex psychosomatic influences on humans. It is proposed that sound is perceived through hearing, through the skin and the sound sensitive parts of skin: the Pacinian corpuscles, as well as acupuncture points connected with acupuncture channels, organs, tissues and cells. Each part of the acoustic system generates different responses after sound, including complex nervous and hormonal reactions, emotional responses, secondary physiological reactions (changes in activity of blood pressure, heart rate, breathing) and pain reduction. (*Sergey Shushardzhan*)

reframing

Changing the musical background or musical environment to alter the orientation of the client's playing. During music play, the *mt* changes their music to reorient the music of the client(s) when the client's music remains consistent or static. As a result, the client's music can take on a new role and relationship to the music and the therapist. (*Kalani Das*)

regulative music therapy (RMT)

A receptive MT approach first developed by Christoph Schwabe (2007) in Germany in the 1960s as individual therapy, later developed as group MT. The theoretical background of RMT is Frankl's logotherapy (paradoxical intention), behaviour therapy (treating symptoms like anxiety) and deep psychology (becoming conscious of defence mechanisms). RMT has six steps. A complete process of all six steps typically requires a minimum of 50 sessions. In the end of the first three steps a client can describe 10 minutes very detailed a two-second interval of his or her perception of music, thoughts, emotions and body. In the next three steps, clients identify individually not accepted perceptions and reduce selection mechanisms of perceiving these. Finally, clients apply this new competence in everyday situations. Final steps review desensitization (behaviour therapy) and mindfulness. Contraindications to RMT are psychotic disorders. Research outcomes of RMT showed best results in group therapy in treatment of anxiety symptoms and somatoform disorders and in individual therapy for borderline personality disorder and eating disorders (Wosch, 2007; Roehrborn, 2007). (*Thomas Wosch*)

relational rehabilitation

An emerging perspective and theoretical base for relational rehabilitation is built on the ideology of an individual situated in their partnerships, family, society and culture. As an example, in the case of health care following traumatic brain injury, relational neurorehabilitation resists an inward search for isolated brain function that can be stimulated remotely and turns outwards to consider the effects of the brain injury upon the relational and social actions and interactions within the client's family and social relationships (Bowen, Yates and Palmer, 2010). Relational rehabilitation provides a conceptual framework for MT practices (Gilbertson and Aldridge, 2008) and draws on contemporary neuroscience that advances the theoretical basis of the social brain (Cozolino, 2006) and the extended mind (Clark, 2008). (*Simon Gilbertson*)

relationship completion

A model of MT practice in palliative care developed by Dileo and Dneaster (2005), Dileo and Loewy (2005) and expanded upon by Clements-Cortés (2004) that includes three levels of practice: supportive (palliative end-of-life symptoms like pain, comfort, quality of life); communicative/expressive (for example, launching and reflective techniques, musical autobiographies, improvisation); transformative (such as life review, resolving conflicts and feelings, addressing spiritual issues). Relationships include the intrapersonal, interpersonal, and/or transpersonal. (*Kevin Kirkland*)

relaxation

Typically receptive MT method that can be used as a technique within a session or as a component of other methods such as in guided imagery and music (Grocke and Wigram, 2007b). Relaxation inductions incorporate live or recorded music and can be administered to a variety of clinical settings. The use of music in progressive muscle relaxation, for example, may enhance a client's attention to task (Robb, 2000). There are many therapeutic benefits to relaxation including breath regulation, pain, anxiety and stress reduction, improved cognitive clarity and enhanced wellbeing (Grocke and Wigram, 2007). An innovative approach to relaxation in MT is Thane's (2011) vocal-led relaxation for children with autism, which aims to develop self-awareness and a mind–body connection (Thane, 2011). In this method, 'the voice is supported by the piano, and it is their marriage and interplay that delivers the therapeutic content' (p. 45). (*Esther Thane*)

religion

A set of beliefs that conveys a particular understanding of the truth surrounding human existence and experience, as well as the existence of divine beings responsible for creation. Faith is expressed through specific devotions and rituals practised by groups of people, or sects, of the same faith. Each sect's dogma, or moral codes and rules for human conduct, are taught by designated persons within an established institution. Music and other art forms often play a central role in faith expression. The role of religion in MT, as well as its links to and distinctions from the concept of spirituality, is an important and ongoing discussion among *mts*. David Aldridge (2003) writes: '...if spirituality is about the individual, ineffable and implicit, religion is about the social, spoken and explicit.' (n.p.) In other words, religious beliefs and practices outwardly express elements of an individual's spiritual essence, and can help the individual find hope, purpose and meaning to help relieve suffering. 'It is in the understanding of suffering, the universality of suffering and the need for deliverance from it that varying traditions of music therapy and religion meet.' (Aldridge, 2003: n.p.) *(Shirley Khalil)*

reminiscence

'A naturally occurring process of recalling personally experienced events' (Webster and McCall, 1999: 73) and (Bohlmeijer *et al.,* 2007) an important part of successful aging, providing a sense of psychosocial wellbeing, enhancing meaning, preserving a sense of mastery and reintegrating unfulfilled dreams; a five-step protocol (Lin, Dai and Hwang, 2003) attempts to make the intervention more standardized; *mts* facilitate reminiscence, stimulating memories through engagement with music of special meaning to the client, evoking thoughts and feelings. For people with Alzheimer's disease (Guétin *et al.,* 2012), therapeutic objectives include enhancing short- and long-term memory processes, encouraging autobiographical memories and preserving identity. Ashida (2000) suggests that reminiscence MT may reduce depressive symptoms in the elderly with dementia, creating opportunities for interpersonal interactions and improving self-image. Reminiscence can be used as a part of the more in-depth therapy process of life review (Cadrin, 2006; Gallagher *et al.,* 2006; Somody, 2010). When communication difficulties interfere with processing, because of cognitive disability (Cevasco, 2010) or language (Grocke and Ip-Winfield, 2011), it is important to be sensitive to client needs, especially when music may trigger unpleasant memories. Although literature focuses on end-of-life issues, *mts* also use reminiscence in work with caregivers (Hanser *et al.,* 2011) and children with traumatic brain injury (Gilbertson, 2009). (*Robin Rio*)

repetition

The major aspect of creating music and an important parameter in achieving therapeutic goals in MT treatment. Repeated content makes patterns which facilitate the application of MT techniques. These patterns are not only processed as a structural entity but also 'heard' within the context of past listening experiences that have contributed to the development of neural networks and associations (Gfeller *et al.,* 2003). As a result of repetition, the listeners might have developed familiarity with the music stimuli, which could support efficacy of the treatment (Lim, 2010). (*Ivana Ilic*)

resistance

A paradoxical, often unconscious, behaviour that serves to undermine a client's therapeutic goals. Resistance is commonly employed as a defence against fear of unpleasant emotions and experiences associated with the past. Forms of resistance in MT may include missed therapy sessions and reluctance to playing or responding to music. For additional information on resistance in MT clients and therapists, see Austin and Dvorkin (1993). Resistance on the part of the *mt* is usually termed as countertransference. (*Paul Nolan*)

resource-oriented music therapy (ROMT)

Rolvsjord (2010) offered a conceptual framework for ROMT based on four relational stances: 1) nurturing strengths, resources, and potentials; 2) collaborating rather than intervening; 3) viewing the individual as part of a context; and 4) using music as a resource. ROMT as a political stance challenges static views of illness and treatment in favour of participatory, discursive engagements with music in health care. (*Simon Gilbertson*)

rhythm and motor skills

Rhythm is the organization of time and movement in music. Such movement is organized in three basic ways: 1) tempo (the speed at which a series of beats moves along); 2) pulse (the grouping of beats into units of stressed and unstressed sound; 3) quality (the particular movement effects caused by a variety of rhythmic device) (Ratner, 1966). Rhythm is an essential component of most music. When the music from all cultures of the world is considered, rhythm is often most fundamental. Krumhansl (2000) said that rhythm is the organizer and the energizer. Rhythm can increase range of motion and repertoire of motor patterns and maintain muscle function and increase motor coordination in clients who have orthopaedic impairments (Miller, 1979). Rhythm can be used to enhance the structure of a motor training programme for learning disability clients who have difficulties with spatial perception. (*Ali Zadeh Mohammadi*)

rhythm and the internal body

Synchronization of physiological rhythms of the body (heart frequency, pulse, brain waves) and external rhythmical stimuli created through live or recorded music, particularly influenced by tempo. The *mt* can obtain a specific physiological effect by matching the client's pulse to the music and subsequently influence the pulse in the desired direction, a technique based on Altshuler's (1948) ISO principle. Rider (1997, 1999) has developed a therapeutic procedure on this principle combined with a theory called homeodynamics or Trevarthen's (2009) biochronology. Music can closely correlate to body rhythms, providing a unique interface between sensations evoked in the mind with other neurological events.

Music can function to bypass other areas of the brain which may be damaged or develop pathways to underdeveloped areas; and can organize events in a global way (Pavlicevic, 1997). (*Ali Zadeh Mohammadi*)

Robbins, Carol (1942–1996)

Music therapist, music educator and composer, Carol held Bachelor's and Master's degrees in music education, certification in special education and an honorary Doctorate of Humane Letters from Potsdam College at the State University of New York. Carol specialized in music education with the deaf and hard of hearing when she began studying with Paul Nordoff and Clive Robbins in 1966. She married Clive in 1975 and worked with him on a music curriculum development programme at the New York State School for the Deaf. They wrote a comprehensive curriculum guide, *Music for the hearing impaired and other special groups* (Robbins and Robbins, 1980). Later, they worked as a team to continue the development of Nordoff–Robbins MT. Carol worked clinically, lectured and gave seminars, workshops and training courses internationally. In 1989, Carol and Clive returned to the USA to establish and co-direct the Nordoff–Robbins Center for Music Therapy at New York University. She received a number of honours and awards. Carol's voice and piano skills were powerful tools in her work with children with disabilities and on her tremendous influence as a teacher of *mts*. Carol died of cancer in 1996 at the age of 54. Her work and music live on through numerous songs that she improvised and composed while working with children, which are now published in various venues (Nordoff *et al.,* 1995; Ritholz and Robbins, 1999, 2003; Robbins and Robbins, 1991a, 1991b; Robbins, 1997). (*Barbara Wheeler*)

Robbins, Clive (1927–2011)

Clive began his work as a special education teacher in 1954 at Sunfield Children's Home in the Midlands of England, a Steiner community for children with multiple challenges, later describing it as 'the first profoundly fulfilling experience of my life' (Telegraph, 2012). With composer Paul Nordoff, they co-founded Nordoff–Robbins Music Therapy in 1959 (Robbins, 2005). They collaborated from 1959 to 1974 (Nordoff–Robbins Center for Music Therapy, 2013). Clive collaborated with his wife, Carol Robbins, from 1975 onwards (Aigen *et al.,* 2007). Clive was 'closely involved in developing centers for the practice, study, and research of the N–R approach in the United Kingdom, Germany, Australia, Japan, Korea, and the United States' (Robbins, 2005: back cover). He was the Founding Director of the Nordoff-Robbins Center for MT at New York University. (*Jennifer Lin*)

rock music

'Rock-n-Roll' was first used by Alan Freed in 1951 (Shaw, 1986). Rock began as a fusion of rhythm 'n' blues, pop and country-and-western musical elements

(Southern, 1997). The music is characterized by small combos (groups) of musicians (Shaw, 1986). Although other instruments can often be heard, the instrumentation of rock ensembles typically includes bass guitar, drum set and electric guitar (Shaw, 1986). Rhythmic complexity is one of the most important musical characteristics in this style of music (Wicke, 1991). Rock music typically emphasizes the layering of short rhythmic motifs played by the various instruments, with an emphasis on the backbeat, the second and fourth beats in a 4/4 time signature (Wicke, 1991). (*Peter Meyer*)

rondo

A musical form based on an A-B-A-C-A-D-A pattern. After establishment of a theme, (A), a change, (B), is introduced, followed by return to the original theme, (A), or a close variant. In improvisation, the rondo provides a grounded structure for musical creativity, exploration and dissonance that may culminate or resolve in a safe return home to a central, recurring theme (Wigram, 2004: 205). (*Kevin Kirkland*)

Ruppenthal, Wayne (1913–1997)

Wayne 'Rupe' Ruppenthal was born in Russell, Kansas. As a boy, he listened to Chicago Radio broadcasts of jazz greats and formed a dance band in the seventh grade. He attended the University of Kansas off and on for 14 years, eventually earning a degree in music education, as well as their first Master's degree in MT in 1948. He subsequently held the position of Director of MT for the Topeka State Hospital for 20 years. He maintained an active career as a prominent freelance jazz musician, combining his work with music performances at a variety of venues, radio broadcasts and bands of all kinds (Leisenring, 2001). 'His contributions to the profession were significant and enduring and included establishing formal clinical practice and training standards, assisting with development of the NAMT and promoting the credibility of MT through published research. He retired from Topeka State Hospital in 1968' (Miller, 1999: 105). (*Kevin Kirkland*)

Ruud, Even (b. 1947)

Norwegian *mt*, musicologist, psychologist, researcher and educator who first trained as a piano teacher in Norway and later went on to become a trained *mt* in the USA. He received a PhD with a dissertation on MT from the University of Oslo, where he is currently employed as Professor in the Department of Musicology. He is also Adjunct Professor at Aalborg University and Norges Musikkhøgskole. Ruud has been a key influence in MT education in Norway and abroad since 1978. He has authored more than 15 books and his publications have been translated into many languages. Major English publications include his works from 1980, 1997, 1998 and 2010. (*Lars Ole Bonde*)

scope of practice

Concise description of activities and areas of practice developed for a profession. Such description is informed by the education requirements within a profession, core knowledge and competencies associated with a discipline and expectations for ethical conduct and standards of behaviour in public service. Scope of practice statements are essential for developing and maintaining practitioner training requirements, employee hiring guidelines and ensuring the integrity of the profession as a whole. Nonetheless, scope of practice statements within the same profession may vary within and across organizational jurisdictions and geographical boundaries, based on shifting and subtle understandings of practice. In MT, a scope of practice is typically determined by a therapist's training, descriptions and standards adopted by educators, healthcare providers, professional organizations and regulatory bodies, as well as by client needs in a particular work environment. Scope of practice statements are intended to define the parameters of MT to other healthcare professionals and *mts*, as well as clients, employers, courts and educators, with a view to inform the public about professional MT services. (*Kevin Kirkland*)

Sears, William W. (1922–1980)

MT professor, theoretician, researcher and tuba player, Bill Sears served as drum major of the University of Kansas band in 1941–43 and 1946–48. He won the national baton-twirling championship at the Chicagoland Music Festival at Soldier Field in 1942 and 1948. After finishing his undergraduate music education degree in 1947, he studied MT at Kansas with E. Thayer Gaston and served as the first research assistant in the newly organized laboratory for the investigation of the influence of music on behaviour. His early research focused on physiological responses to music stimuli. He was the first editor of the *Journal of Music Therapy* (1964–67) and served as President of the NAMT (1971–73). His influential theoretical chapter, 'Processes of music therapy', appeared in Gaston's *Music in therapy* (1968). His teaching career included Washburn University (1955–57), Ohio University (1957–63), Indiana University (1963–68) and the University of Kansas (1968–80). Sears played national leadership roles in professional organizations, including the NAMT, the Music Educators National Conference, the Music Teachers National Association. He presented many programmes at national and regional meetings of these groups. His widow, Margaret Sears, published a collection of his writings (Sears, 2007). (*George Duerksen*)

self-experience

Awareness of one's experience from the first-person perspective. Although it is not clear yet in current research whether the identification of something as oneself as distinguished from others is necessary for self-experience, its bodily roots and the existence of pre-linguistic forms of self-awareness have been acknowledged. In neonate and infant therapy, empathy is considered to be a form of self-experience related to others in the course of pursuits and relations (Lysaker and Lysaker, 2010). (*Jin Hyun Kim*)

self-inquiry

Sometimes spelled self-enquiry, it belongs to the tradition of heuristic research and is a method of exploring personal experiences, prejudices and tacit knowledge. It often begins with a personal question or challenge that has a social or universal significance. The life experience or assumptions of the heuristic or phenomenological or hermeneutic researcher and the research participants is studied as more or less focused and comprehensive stories that can also be further elucidated through art and personal documentations. From these individual depictions and portraits from research participants, a composite depiction is developed and the primary researcher then develops a creative synthesis from this material. In MT research, the tradition is also called first-person research (Bruscia, 2005) and it may include the use of personal construct theory (Abrams and Meadows, 2005). Self-inquiry can be a self-awareness tool for researcher or *mt*; a means of controlled subjectivity (Smeijsters, 2005a; Roberts, 2003). Self-inquiry allows the researcher to explore and explicate their attitudes, judgments, beliefs, emotions, thoughts and reactions related to any facet of a research study. In clinical work, it allows for the *mt* to explore episodes of countertransference (Bruscia, 1995). Self-inquiry techniques can be experiential (for example, improvising, creating mandalas) or reflective (such as journaling, seeking supervision, doing meditative exercises or writing a musical autobiography chronicling the occurrence and significance of music experiences throughout various stages of life) (Bruscia, 1998c). (*Lars Ole Bonde and Julie Lytle*)

sensorial play

A term describing the characteristic playing of a client where, while producing sounds, the client is not able to connect with or experience these sounds as being self-produced (De Backer, 2005). The client's music is characterized by repetitiveness and/or fragmentation. The improvisation cannot really be begun nor ended and there is no clear melodic, rhythmic or harmonic development, no variation and no recapitulation; the client is perceptually and emotionally detached from their musical production. Therefore, improvising is not a real 'experience' for the client; it is not inspired or affected by the music and remains disconnected from the sounds and the playing. There is an absence of shared playing and inter-subjectivity with the *mt*, in the sense that the client does not engage in the joint music creation. In terms of the psychopathology of psychotic or autistic clients, one can say they cannot create a psychic space that allows symbolization (Van Camp and De Backer, 2012), thus making it impossible for them to produce appropriate musical material. The *mt* experiences the client as isolated and becomes completely caught up in the client's music and is not free to introduce musical images and, because of this, no interaction is possible in the 'co-play'. (*Jos De Backer*)

sensory cortex

The portion of the brain responsible for processing all tactile input. Also known as the somatosensory cortex, the sensory cortex is located directly behind (posterior to) the central sulcus of the cerebral cortex. The sensory cortex of each hemisphere processes tactile input from the opposite side of the body. The conscious sense of touch is thought to originate in the somatosensory cortex (Meyer 2011). Adjacent areas of the body are represented by adjacent areas of the sensory cortex; this 'map' of the body is known as the sensory homunculus. Sensory cortex can also be used in a much broader sense to describe all of the sensory processing areas, including the somatosensory cortex, visual cortex, auditory cortex, primary olfactory cortex and gustatory cortex) (FitzGerald, 2012). Playing an instrument sends tactile messages to the sensory cortex (Gaidos, 2010: 27). (*Charles Limb and Malinda McPherson*)

sensory integration

The neurological process that organizes sensation(s) from one's sensory systems as well as the environment, sensory integration was initially introduced into the occupational therapy literature by Ayers (1979), then subsequently brought into the special education literature by Greenspan and Weider (1998), and then to MT for both individuals (Berger, 2002) and group members (Goodman, 2007) to help *mts* to understand the importance of modulating sensory input, particularly for the client with sensory integration dysfunction. Sensory inputs are perceived by sensory receptors and connected to the reticular activating system to regulate arousal reactions within the central nervous system (CNS). All these stimuli travel through the CNS to the brain, flowing along the spinal cord, brain stem, paleoencephalon and neocortex. Next, they are decoded and transformed in responses for assuring safety and well being at subcortical level, afterward in cognitive and psychological meanings at neocortical level (Schneck and Berger, 2006). Since sound stimuli can be configured before a neocortex processing, the music proceeds directly in the paleoencephalon (through the limbic system) and can engage clients with sensory disorders, mental health needs or developmental and learning disabilities. (*Claudio Cominardi and Karen Goodman*)

sexual identity

Self-recognition of one's sexual orientation and behaviour that influence individuals' perceptions of themselves on the spectrum as heterosexual, gay, lesbian, bisexual or transgendered. A person's sexual identity may or may not be congruent with sexual orientation and behaviour and can change over time. Incongruence between sexual identity and sexual behaviour may, for example, reflect a particular culture's way of understanding sexuality (Rust, 2003), given that sexuality is often viewed as socially and culturally constructed. Sexual identity differs from gender identity, which refers to an individual's view of self as male, female or intersex; this may or may not correspond to their biological gender or designated sex at birth. (*Bill Ahessy*)

Sharpe, Norma (1907–1996)

One of the first *mts* working independently in Canada in the 1950s, together with Fran Herman and Thérèse Pageau. In 1960, Sharpe conducted a survey of music in hospitals across Canada, discovering that only three of 49 musical staff were trained *mts*. This survey provided a baseline measure for *mts* and increased its awareness in hospitals and institutions. By the 1970s, Sharpe had regular contact with 300 individuals and organizations across Canada sharing an interest in this emerging field. In 1974, she presided over the first MT conference at St Thomas Psychiatric Hospital in St Thomas, Ontario, with the theme 'Music therapy: an idea whose time has come'. The enthusiasm of the 63 delegates set the foundation for MT as a valuable contributor to Canadian health care. According to Sharpe (1977), that first conference was organized to unify personnel who were working in MT throughout Canada, to become aware of one another's existence and to share techniques, programmes and assessment of rehabilitative effectiveness. (*Kevin Kirkland*)

silence

Silence marks the beginning and ending of a sound experience. Juliette Alvin believed that, for clients to feel sound, they needed to discover silence as its counterpart: 'music or sound emerges from silence and returns to silence' (Alvin, 1966: 287). Her words highlight the need for spaces that invite silence between, during and after an MT session. Silence may be a fertile space to refocus and redirect creativity or a space of self-reflection, contemplation and illumination. The therapist or client who is uncomfortable with silence might fill every musical or spoken moment; therefore, silence may be used to facilitate or obstruct therapeutic goals and interventions. Silence may also present itself as hardened resistance, a protective shell against participation in the therapeutic process. (*Kevin Kirkland*)

single-case research design

In MT single-case research, a single individual or group is treated as their own control, thus eliminating the need for a control group. To account for as many passage-of-time-related threats to internal validity as possible, single-case designs observe the subject/participant in both control and (single or multiple) treatment conditions, alternating or randomizing the order of these conditions to determine whether cause-and-effect relationships exist between independent and dependent variables. Commonly used designs include: partial and full reversal designs (e.g. A-B-A, A-B-A-B), multiple baseline designs across subjects, behaviours or settings; multiple treatment designs; alternating/multiple conditions/treatment designs, and others. Qualitative single-case research often involves careful and repeated observation of an individual or group in a naturalistic setting, gathering rich data through observation, self-report and artefacts such as recorded music, video or interviews. Quantitative single-case designs allow the researcher to statistically or visually compare numerical results of how the subject performs under different circumstances (baseline and one or more treatment conditions). Visual analysis of data points via graphing may provide evidence of change in dependent variables if the data often do not meet the requirements for parametric statistics. (*Robert Krout*)

slide guitar

Refers to a style of playing guitar, credited to being developed by Joseph Kekuku (Mann, 1996) and can be heard in many different genres such as country, blues, rock and folk (James, 1999). The technique involves placing a firm object such as a comb, knife, or bottle, on the strings and sliding it from one note to the next (Meyer, De Villers and Ebnet, 2010). Although chords can be played with a slide in standard tuning, the guitar is often tuned to an open chord to make the task easier (Mann, 1996). It can serve as an adaptive way of playing guitar, as the style requires little hand strength and fret markers make it easy to know where to place the slide (Meyer, De Villers and Ebnet, 2010). (*Peter Meyer*).

social justice

A concept that emphasizes a society founded on principles of equality, one that values and promotes human rights regardless of country of origin, economic status, race, religion, sexual orientation, and so on. According to Amnesty International, human rights not only include 'freedom of expression and freedom from torture and ill-treatment, but also rights to education, to adequate housing and other economic, social and cultural rights' (Amnesty International, 2011). Engaging in social justice involves more than consciousness-raising: it involves actively working to eliminate structural injustices based upon one group or individual having unfair power or privilege over another group or individual. A significant issue for *mts* concerned with social justice is to address the problem of health inequities within and between countries and to examine the ways in which we support these inequities by placing greater resources into individualized treatment versus community and public health practices. In MT, social justice is a major focus in feminist MT, community MT and for groups such as Music Therapists for Peace. (*Susan Hadley*)

sociocultural theories

The family of theories based on the pioneering cultural historical psychology of Lev Vygotsky and other Russian psychologists of the early twentieth century is often called sociocultural theories and includes traditions such as activity theory and cultural psychology. Related theory traditions exist within anthropology, sociology and other disciplines. Contemporary sociocultural theories focus on the interplay and reciprocal influence between individual actions and culturally organized activities. The entity of study is the individual in context but the individual is not seen as a product of context. Instead, there is focus on the transactional processes between the individual and the milieu. Sociocultural theories include but go beyond biological and psychological perspectives; a basic idea is that human nature demands social nurture mediated by cultural artefacts to develop. The sociocultural perspective also invites investigations of how culture and mind make up each other, over the history of communities and over the life course of the individual. Culture-centred MT can be considered a member of the family of sociocultural theories (Stige, 2002a), as it is a perspective that highlights music as social participation nurtured by cultural history, the history of the species and the history of the individual. (*Brynjulf Stige*)

sociometric evaluation

A method of evaluation in MT in which clients are administered a sociometric questionnaire requiring them to rank other group members on an affective or friendship criterion such as: Who is the most entertaining? Who is the most popular? Who is the most accomplished? The questionnaire analysis yields clinical data such as group cohesiveness (number of reciprocal choices), stars (most choices), isolates (unchosen) and peer acceptance (a client's cumulative rank position in the group). Sociometry was developed by Austrian psychiatrist and philosopher J. L. Moreno (1889–1974), adapted for use in MT to examine group dynamics (Braswell *et al.,* 1970) and to effectively evaluate the results of MT activities (Cassity, 1976, 1981). (*Michael Cassity*)

song circle

Also called soulsong circle. An *a cappella* vocal improvisation technique used to playfully explore sounds, feelings, role relationships, and more. In this technique, adapted for therapeutic use by Virginia Schenck (personal communication, 8 February 2012), musical elements (such as tempo, pitch, timbre, melody harmony, rhythm, meter and dynamics) are applied, layered and manipulated to create soundscapes. In a basic application of this technique, the song leader establishes an ostinato that is continued by a portion of the circle. Additional vocal patterns are assigned to other sections of the circle until everyone is engaged in the vocalization. Because of the improvisatory nature of song circles, sounds can be modified, layers created or removed, and solos may be sung spontaneously over the other vocalizations. Words are not required and, when used, need not make sense. Vocables or scat singing (sung syllables that have no conscious meaning) are often preferred for the freedom they represent and the fun of making the sounds (Schmidt-Jones, 2011; V. Schenck, personal communication, 8 February 2012). The process of leading a song circle or improvising a part may be integral to the therapeutic process for some clients. Song circles for therapeutic use were developed as a result of Schenck's work with Bobby McFerrin (1997) in CircleSongs and improvisation with Rhiannon, a member of McFerrin's *Voicestra*. (*Rebecca Engen*)

song collage

The use of words and phrases from existing songs as part of the lyric formation process in creating therapeutically oriented songs (Tamplin, 2006). The *mt* supports the client to review lyrics from songbooks or the inserts of compact discs to gain ideas for what they might want to include in their own song composition. Words or specific lyrics may speak to the client, representing or reflecting their context, feelings, ideas or experiences. These identified song fragments are meshed together to form a song – a collage. The client may add additional material. This technique is particularly useful for people who have intellectual, emotional, congenital or acquired neurological challenges around identifying their thoughts and feelings. For them, it may be easier to have insight into their situation when reviewing other songwriters' lyrics. Similarly, cognitive challenges may limit the clients' abilities to initiate or generate ideas to integrate into the song lyrics. (*Felicity Baker*)

song histories

The story or origins behind how a song came to be written, the life experiences of the author, the inspiration for the lyrics, the origins of the melody, the culture, context and era of when the song was written, all make for opportunities for reminiscing, learning and dialogue. Knowing the history behind a song can deepen the appreciation for it and can enhance the emotional connection to it. Sometimes research into the history of a song reveals original lyrics or additional verses. Song histories can also be applied to music without words, where the autobiography and life context of the composer can be shared. The scope of using song histories can be as light as a music appreciation group, the deepening of connection to a higher power through the stories behind sacred songs and hymns, or as rich as songs that speak to challenges clients deal with. (*Kevin Kirkland*)

song of kin

A relevant song or melody that has significance to a person and when shared can initiate or deepen a therapeutic relationship. The music of a kin (Loewy, 2000) is an orienting theme, which accompanies a client through transformation(s). The song of kin may be relevant to one's culture, either from religious affiliation, early childhood, or may be a melody that is referentially significant or simply passed down from one's familial line from one generation to the next. Its function is similar to the term, contact song. (*Joanne Loewy*)

song parody

One of a number of therapeutic song writing approaches whereby the lyrics of a pre-composed song chosen by the therapist and/or client are replaced by the client's own words. Clinicians may choose this approach when: the pre-existing song expresses an emotion, situation, issue or story that resonates with that of the client's; when the client's musical identity is strongly represented in the pre-existing song and it is therefore therapeutically important to reinforce this; if the client's cognitive or communication skills are more suited to song parody than freely composed songs; or when time available to create songs is limited. Song parody can be done individually or with a group. (*Felicity Baker*)

song stories, improvised *see* improvised song stories

sound

A perception caused by mechanical vibrations that are transmitted through an elastic medium (solid, liquid or gas). Sound frequencies are located within a scale range of 20–20,000 Hz. When the sound pressure is higher than 20 μP (micropascals) it becomes detectable to human ears (Jauset, 2010). These vibrations produce variations on different atmospheric pressure levels that are converted into electronic impulses when reaching the auditory system. The impulses are transmitted through to the thalamus into the auditory cortex by the auditory nerve where the information is decoded into a sensation called sound. This is a very complex process that involves several brain areas belonging to both hemispheres. It may be said that sound only exists within the brain (Izquierdo, Oliver and Malmierca, 2009). (*Jordi A. Jauset*)

sound duet

Priestley (1994) defines a difference between our relationships through words compared with our musical relationships. In the music or sound expression, we are more immediately responsive and in connection with the client's feelings and expression. The therapist and client, through co-creating this sound duet, can reflect upon all that can be heard and felt in the experience. Recording can allow for improved processing opportunities. From this merger within the music, the therapist and client can therapeutically separate in their analysis of the recording, re-enacting the symbiosis and healthy separation/individuation referred to in child development theories (Winnicott, 1971/1997; Schiff and Schiff, 1971;

Kohut and Levarie, 1950) and often applicable to adults recovering from unhealthy beginnings. 'We part', said Priestley, 'as separate beings' (Priestley and Eschen, 2002: 13). (*Kevin Kirkland*)

speech/language

Complex, temporally varying signals composed of many different acoustic and linguistic properties that may be used for communicating and understanding intended messages (Fogerty and Humes, 2012). Both music and speech/language involve complex and meaningful sound sequences that naturally invite comparisons between the two (Patel, 2008). Owing to similarities between these two categories in their physical and cognitive processing, perception and production, MT interventions such as lyrics, rhythmic work, turn taking, and Melodic Intonation Therapy can be beneficial for clients with speech/language impairments (Leung, 2008). (*Ivana Ilic*)

spirituality

Owing to its highly subjective, contextual and interpretative nature, there is no commonly accepted definition of spirituality. Magill (2006: 173) suggests that, 'spirituality is the concern with acquiring or maintaining an existential way to view and live one's life at a deeper and more meaningful level, and to search for an understanding of the purpose of their joys, trials and sufferings. [...] and is the search for connectedness with self, others and that which lies beyond'. Compared with religion, spirituality involves humans' search for meaning in life without to necessarily involve an organized entity with rituals and practices about a higher power or god(s) (Aldridge, 2006). The significance of spiritual considerations is evident in the work of various MT pioneers (such as Bonny, Nordoff and Robbins) and within the context of different approaches to MT (for example, anthroposophical MT, GIM and creative MT). Some recurring spiritual themes in MT literature include: 1) transcendence and transformation; 2) meaning, purpose and identity in life; 3) faith and hope; and 4) connectedness with self, others and with the sacred/divine or god(s). (*Giorgos Tsiris*)

splitting

Mary Priestley (Priestley and Eschen, 2002) developed the technique of splitting, especially useful where the client has projected part of themselves on to another person and, in doing so, lost the emotion invested in that person. For example, a female client had a domineering father and is now afraid to express anger and has high anxiety in dealing with her male boss, unaware that her reaction to him sparks similar feelings of incompetence and insecurity she felt with her dad. The relationship dynamics can be processed on non-verbal or paraverbal levels through sound expression: the client plays self on their choice of instrument, the *mt* plays how the father would sound (as described or previously portrayed musically by the client). The improvised musical dialogue can open up awareness and affect. Roles can then be switched, wherein it can be very useful for the client to hear how they sound in comparison to the other. This technique can also be used between polarized states, such as angry/polite, hope/despair, parent/child, or other concepts that are black and white or rigidly held. (*Kevin Kirkland*)

standards of practice

Many healthcare professions abide by these and some MT associations also include them with their bylaws and code of ethics. Standards of practice (or practice standards) are used 'where theory meets practice and ethics gain meaning' (CFA Institute, 2005: v). Standards of practice call for a set of guidelines for providing excellence in client-centred MT and criteria for evaluating it. From a legal perspective as applicable in some areas, the standards can be important where a dispute arises over the quality of MT provided. (*Kevin Kirkland*)

story

The powerful oral tradition of conveying experience through imaginative renderings is at the root of story. Stories benefit from a 'Once upon a time' telling, yet also offer powerful here-and-now performances where the client can participate in the unfolding of a tale that is mythical, magical, or factual (Silverman, 2004). The representation of story can be enhanced by musical accompaniment, sounds as symbols of events or characters, dance, drawings, photographs and images and drama. Story is also often encountered in musical lyrics. Instrumental music can relate a story: a beginning, a journey, relationships, difficulties, movement, unexpected surprises, lament and a satisfying conclusion. A song-as-story can have the chorus rewritten, a verse added, the song retitled. It offers the opportunity to re-stor(e)y through talking about the character in the song without – as may sometimes be necessary – talking directly about the clients. Questions for the character: what happened that the person feels this way? What advice would you give? What happens next in their life? In improvisation a therapeutic story, perhaps with elements of Campbell's archetypal hero's journey (Campbell, 1973; Campbell and Moyers, 1988), can provide meaningful rehearsal for life skills. (*Kevin Kirkland and Nancy McMaster*)

Storycomposing®

A model of musical interaction developed by Hakomäki (2009) which provides an opportunity to express feelings and experiences that have significance for clients. The concept of Storycomposing (originally *Tarinasäveltäminen*, in Finnish) developed while working with children under school age in a daycare centre in 1999–2002. The developing process of Storycomposing was carried out listening to and consulting with children. Notation is used to fix the improvised musical creations of clients so that the material can be revisited in future sessions and performed to selected groups of people. No musical talent or prior studies of music are needed. Various ways of notating the scores can be used. Storycomposing is a therapeutic song-writing method influenced by clinical improvisation. The Storycomposing procedure has four steps: 1) musical expression; 2) interaction; 3) a story composition; 4) a performance. Storycomposing is suitable for clients and families aged three and upwards, and for special needs children and adults, psychiatric conditions and dementia. It is also applicable to music education settings, with other creative activities and for supervision. (*Hanna Hakomäki*)

strength-based improvisation

An advanced training course developed by Jackert and Rio (2007) for *mts* in varying stages of professional practice desiring a safe space to improvise with *mt* peers and to explore relational musicality with the aim of advancing clinical musicianship and personal growth. Strengths refers to the clinician working from a place of perceived musical strength by using voice or instrument of choice, rather than a specific musical technique or instrument, in an effort to face fear and discomfort with the unknown elements of improvisation. The *mt* then expands from this place of strength to use music in an interdependent way with a small community of peers to explore areas of perceived weakness. Extended improvisational musical play, musical autobiography, peer supervision, movement, creative arts and elements of playback theatre are used to enhance the group process. (*Robin Rio*)

success oriented

Focuses on the clients' abilities rather than their areas of deficit. In success-oriented practices, the *mt* will set a number of challenging, yet achievable, objectives for the client, so that they can meet their overarching goal. In this regard, it may be considered more challenging than failure-free activities. By focusing and challenging a clients' strengths and abilities, the client can gain skills and confidence, which in turn may be generalized to other aspects of the client's life. (*Naomi Bell*)

supervision

An intensive, interpersonally focused relationship in which a supervisor is designated to facilitate and promote the development of therapeutic competence and effectiveness of the supervisee (Hawkins and Shohet, 2000; Loganbill, Hardy and Delworth, 1982) within a mutual collaboration context. MT supervision aims for an open and honest articulation of material arising from the work upon musical, practical or dynamic issues, within a supportive, critically reflective and analytical framework (Bunt and Hoskyns, 2002). Thereby, supervision becomes an ongoing process of the working practice in which both supervisor and supervisee constantly interact through examination and exploration of casework (Forinash, 2001). Supervision enables the supervisee to develop knowledge, understanding, ideas and self-observation skills within a safe, protective space, not only for their own benefit but also for protecting the client's best interests (Hawkins and Shohet, 2000). Supervision may also involve inter-professional, ethical or administrative issues in a work setting, as well as peer discussion, experiential music and role-playing, team interaction, reflections on feelings within the clinical process, monitoring and evaluation of practice (Odell-Miller and Richards, 2009). There are various practical and theoretical approaches that may emphasize different aspects depending on the MT methods used, theoretical orientation, key issues addressed, stage of professional and personal development of the supervisor and supervisee or cultural dynamics (Hawkins and Shohet, 2000; Odell-Miller and Richards, 2009). (*Evangelia Papanikolaou*)

supportive activity-level music therapy

Wheeler (1983) classified levels of music psychotherapy based on Wolberg's (1977) psychotherapeutic levels. At the supportive or activity level, the *mt* takes a directive role in leading the session and focuses on the development of a positive relationship with the client to help the client to develop adaptive behaviours. The focus is on the use of client resources and achievement of goals through music activities rather than emphasis on the insight, processing, and other analytic devices. (*Lillian Eyre*)

supportive mirroring

Supportively reflecting the client's (often improvised) music by highlighting a therapeutically significant element, quality or aspect (Bruscia, 1987a: 344). It shares similarities with related terms of mirroring and matching. (*Kevin Kirkland*)

supportive psychotherapy

An effective treatment for a broad range of clients and clients; an interpersonal bond which is affectively responsive and focused on here-and-now concerns of the client. A goal is to help clients adapt better to their life and return to the level of functioning in which they were living before the crisis that occurred and which brought them into treatment. For those with persistent mental illness, goals are designed to reduce anxiety, improve reality testing and to help the individual to live more comfortably with their psychopathology. In MT, this method seems to be the default approach taken by *mts* working with psychiatric or medically ill clients. (*Paul Nolan*)

symbolic representation and transformation

A view of the client's music – often during improvisation though also possible through choice of song, instrument, motif, lyrics, listening preferences – as a metaphor or symbol of a symptom or illness (McClary, 2007). By extension, symptom may instead be thought of as an issue, mood, strength, or other metaphor. Applied directly for this purpose, the client is asked to imagine their symptom(s) in musical form, inventing sounds to give their symptom an audible representation. McClary's Jungian approach to MT said that the fusion of symptoms and music allows new possibilities by walking around the experience –circumambulating it – from multiple perspectives. Through processing approaches, such as insights, recognizing patterns, experimenting and meaning making, the client may transcend the symptom, which is musical transformation. (*Kevin Kirkland*)

synchronization

The process of matching an external periodic [having marked or repeated cycles] stimulus, often via physical movement. An ensemble following a conductor is synchronizing with a visual stimulus, while marching to a drum line's pattern is synchronizing with an aural stimulus. Humans readily synchronize to periodicities within the general range of 40–300 beats per minute (Van Noorden and Moelants, 1999), although the boundaries of this range are dependent on many factors, such as the type of physical movement involved, the age of the synchronizer and the presence or absence of other related periodicities in a complex stimulus such as most music. (*Peter Martens*)

systematic reviews

These are conducted using explicit, exhaustive pre-determined search strategies. Quality assessment of included studies is essential in order to achieve rigor in synthesis of the findings. It aims to minimise bias in reviewing research evidence and systematic reviews are particularly popular in health research to review effectiveness of clinical interventions. The use of meta-analysis is common though it is not mandatory. Systematic reviews of randomised controlled studies, for example standard Cochrane Reviews, are regarded as the best evidence in the hierarchical 'levels of evidence' framework at the Centre of Evidence Based Medicine at University of Oxford. Many quantitative systematic reviews are limited when exploring heterogeneity of clinical evidence and this can particularly be problematic when reviewing a complex intervention such as music therapy. The inclusion of qualitative research in systematic reviews has now been widely accepted (Dixon-Woods, 2001). Some traditional narrative reviews have been criticised for the lack of transparency in the selection procedures and in the synthesis method. However, the use of an explicit narrative format, such as

Narrative Synthesis in Systematic Reviews (Popay, 2006), allows systematic evaluations of diverse evidence and increases trustworthiness of the reviews. (*McDermott*)

therapeutic alliance

Refers to the collaborative aspect of the relationship between therapist and client. It is a way of looking at the therapeutic relationship through the lens of effective goal-directed work (Muran and Barber, 2010). Bordin (1979) developed the alliance theory, which indicates three components of the alliance: 1) an agreement between therapist and client about the goals of treatment; 2) an agreement about the therapy tasks needed to accomplish those goals; and 3) the emotional bond developed between therapist and client. The contributors of the alliance theory have highlighted the negotiation process in forming and maintaining the alliance, paying particular attention to the issue of openly and effectively countering the client's disagreement or doubt about the treatment (Safran *et al.,* 2005). If the experience of the client does not meet their expectations, the client will withdraw temporarily or permanently. The technique that feels meaningful and goal-directed and engages the client is the best promoter of good alliance (Muran and Barber, 2010). The quality of the therapeutic relationship influences technique effectiveness (Goldfried and Davila, 2005) and research has shown that a good therapeutic alliance is one of the most consistent predictors of treatment success (Crits-Christoph, Gibbons and Hearon, 2006; DeRubeis, Brotman and Gibbons, 2005; Martin, Garske and Davis, 2000). (*Alice Pehk*)

therapeutic frame

A term used within the psychoanalytic model to delimit the field of work and maintain certain constants: the schedule of care, frequency, length of sessions and fees. Freud (see Pollard, 2004) suggested several ideas to increase the effectiveness of psychoanalysis but made no reference to frame. Winnicott (see Ferraiolo, 2004) was one of the first to use this term. It is also used by some to refer to a setting that includes – besides the constant psychoanalysis – materials, and especially the musical instruments, used during the therapeutic process. The most important use of this term in MT is to outline a framework for the theory in which to develop the musical experience that will help improve a client's quality of life. (*Gabriel Federico*)

therapeutic function of music

The direct relationship between the treatment goal and the explicit characteristics of the musical elements, informed by a theoretical framework and/or philosophical paradigm in the context of a client. (*Deanna Hanson-Abromeit*)

therapeutic intention

This ethical perspective involves having the best interest of the client in mind, especially when the client is not able to articulate or is not fully aware of, their desired goals and needs. Bent Jensen (1999: 45) added, 'There will often be a paradox between the client's explicit needs and the client's 'objective' needs – a paradox between respecting the client's integrity and having the ethical responsibility for the therapy, which includes an ambition of therapeutic change for the patient'. Intention thus includes intervention from a position of best practice and ethical care. (*Kevin Kirkland*)

therapeutic narrative analysis

A flexible research method that helps the therapist to understand the process of therapy. The basis of the analysis are recorded events selected as significant by the researcher as significant and may include both qualitative and quantitative data. At its heart it is hermeneutic; it is based on understanding the meaning of what happens in the process of therapy and therefore naturalistic (Lincoln and Guba, 1985). Central to the narrative methodology is the idea of episodes (Aldridge, 1999; Harré and Secord, 1971). An episode is an event, incident or sequence of events that forms part of a narrative. Therapeutic narratives are composed of episodes and these provide the foundation for the research interpretation. The narrative is the story thread that brings these episodes together over time. We can use a variety of textual materials; written reports, spoken stories, visual media, recorded materials and musical material in the telling of the story. The research part is the analysis of those materials that bring forth new therapeutic understandings, hence therapeutic narrative analysis (Aldridge and Aldridge, 2008). We are able to make explicit the process of interpreting non-verbal materials from the music process itself. (*David Aldridge*)

therapeutic song writing

Involves the client's engagement in the creation, notation, and/or recording of lyrics and music within the context of a therapeutic relationship to address client needs (Wigram and Baker, 2005). The song creations become a tangible record of a client's therapeutic journey or a representation of the client's transformed state. Therapeutic song writing is a suitable intervention across the lifespan and has demonstrated potential to enhance self-confidence and self-esteem, to help develop a sense of self, to assist in externalizing and clarifying thoughts, fantasies and emotions, and to 'tell' the client's story (Baker *et al.*, 2008, 2009). Dependent upon the client's diagnosis and the orientation of the therapist and/or the facility, songs may be created according to principles and practices of: community MT, cognitive behavioural therapy, person-centred therapy, strengths-based approaches and resource-oriented approaches, and may be created in a single session or over several sessions. The process may extend beyond the initial creation, notation and recording; that is, there may be further benefits gained through repeated listening, reflecting and discussing the song's meaning either with the *mt* or through the sharing of the song with others. (*Felicity Baker*)

therapeutic voice work

A broad term used to describe a range of methods that incorporate the use of the voice either by the *mt* and/or by the client/s to achieve a therapeutic change in health and wellbeing, including improved vocal abilities, health and homeostasis and human relationships. According to Uhlig and Baker (2011), voice work involves the use of breath and rhythm, primal sounds of expression and communication building a dialogue between therapist and client/s, using rhythm, intonation, words and fragments of sentences, and offering inter-subjective vocalization (p. 32). Baker and Uhlig (2011) describe a taxonomy of voice-work approaches that include acoustic cueing, contingent singing, dantian respiration, drone, *sori*, sound bath, therapeutic rhythmic chanting, tonal intervallic synthesis, tonal vocal holding and vocal-led relaxation. (*Felicity Baker*)

therapy

Stems from the Greek verb *therapeuin*, meaning to take care of, to heal; the Greek noun *therapeia* meaning service or treatment (Wethered, 1973: x). (*Kevin Kirkland*)

toning

Laurel Keyes introduced to the modern-day world an ancient healing practice called toning. She described it as a process of using 'body-voice' and primordial vocal sounds to release healing energies within the body to effect wholeness and wellbeing (Keyes, 1973: 12). She believed that it was most effective when combined with a specific intent and/or imagery. Subsequent therapists speak about toning as an effective way for 'sound vibrations to free blocked energy and resonate with specific areas of the body to relieve emotional and physical stress and tension' (Austin, 2009: 29). Toning is not singing or chanting. One can do it by and for oneself, with/for another person or in groups. In Austin's vocal psychotherapy work, toning provides a client with immediacy, intimacy, a sensory experience and possibilities of presence and embodiment (p. 31). (*Susan Summers*)

trance

A state of consciousness transformation that can occur during music (Rouget, 1985). Often referred to as a distinct level of consciousness, it is characterized by a restful yet fully alert state of mind with heightened perception, wherein one may experience conflicting perceptions and time shortening (Travis and Pearson, 1999) and a subjectively perceived distortion of the normal spatial relationship between body and mind (Badia, 2001). Balzer (2009) said that trance states can be considered to be elevated forms of states of wellbeing (p. 77). Traditional trance music enhances a feeling of calmness despite the rapid pace of the notes. The constant movement that is repetitious and monotonous creates a secure foundation for this style of music and listening to it is calming for those who enjoy this genre (Grocke and Wigram, 2007a). Ecstasy can result from the resulting stillness and solitude. In the earliest tribes of primitive African cultures, the shaman used music with drum rhythms, bells, special costumes, ritual, text and dance to induce a trance-like state of altered consciousness to achieve crisis resolution and healing (Hamel, 1978; Kovach, 1985). It is easy to overlook the historical use and value of trance states of consciousness evoked from music. It is also important to recognize that such states may be contraindicated for certain populations. Patel (2008) upholds research findings that 'music can play a key role in rapidly transforming the sense of self via an altered states of consciousness known as trance' (p. 324), wherein the trancer enters an altered neurophysiological state. (*Ali Zadeh Mohammadi and Kevin Kirkland*)

transcendence

As a verb, the act of rising above or going beyond the limits of; triumphing over the negative or restrictive aspects of; and extending or lying beyond the limits of ordinary experience. As applied to therapy, transcendence requires a psychological shift in perspective that allows the client to overcome enduring and debilitating aspects of pathology. With this shift in perspective, the client experiences a release from the attendant pathological symptom(s). In MT, music-induced states of altered consciousness are used to promote physical and mental healing, to treat substance dependence and in spiritual and hospice care (Aldridge and Facher, 2006). Examples of this application can be found in GIM practice. To aid the client experiencing transcendence, a GIM programme entitled *Transcendence* was created by Carol Bush and James Borling (Bruscia and Grocke, 2002). Other MT practices employ polyrhythmic music and monotonous drumming to foster transcendence (Aldridge and Facher, 2006). (*Lillian Eyre*)

transformation

A concept associated with transformative learning, based on depth psychology (Boyd and Myers, 1988); applies to therapy in that it indicates a fundamental change in one's personality involving the resolution of a personal dilemma and the expansion of consciousness resulting in greater personality integration (Boyd, in Taylor, 1998: 13). In MT, music is used to evoke symbols, images and archetypes to increase the client's insight leading to expanded consciousness and fundamental change. (*Lillian Eyre*)

transitional object

Winnicott (1953) introduced the term in describing a developmental process with usually takes place for the infant between 4 and 12 months or during the weaning process. This object, discovered or created by the infant, is the first 'not me' possession. It can be a favourite piece of cloth, a stuffed animal or a toy. One of its main functions is to self-soothe and to allow the infant to begin to control inner states of tension during times of stress. The use of the object is the first step toward object relations and later, reality testing. Music, as a transitional object, is demonstrated in the way in which an older child goes over a repertoire of songs and tunes while preparing to go to sleep (Winnicott, 1953: 89). Over time, the object is relied upon less and less but it is still fondly remembered, even into adulthood. In is place, the entire cultural field becomes available, namely, the arts, religion and social groups, among other things and institutions. In MT, Nolan (1989a, 1989b) and Tervo (2005) have published on MT and transitional objects. (*Paul Nolan*)

transpersonal music therapy

Based on the premise that music can transport the client to alternate states of consciousness, transcending the ego and physical body, into spiritual events and what Maslow (1964) would call peak experiences. Such experiences can include the ineffable, altered perception of space and time, intense positive emotion, out-of-body experiences, sense of wholeness or universality, of unity, clarity and understanding. GIM is one possible method, as is free improvisation, group singing/chanting and any other MT experience that promotes a sense of unity and expanded awareness. Integrating spiritual experience within a larger perspective of human nature and development is the aim of transpersonal MT (Crowe, 2004). (*Kevin Kirkland*)

treatment plan

A written document that describes the course of therapeutic intervention. This document provides a narrative overview of the assessment findings and summarizes the client's strengths and needs. Based on this information, subsequent goals and objectives and the method for data collection of those objectives are identified. Proposed MT treatment strategies are described supported by a theoretical framework. (*Cynthia Colwell*)

tuning

The tuning practices of a music tradition govern strong preferences depending on very small differences in pitch; one sound may be perceived as pleasant and correct, while another only a few Hertz lower is perceived as very unpleasant and wrong. There are multiple issues involved; for example: what are the intervals between the correct notes? Are the allowed intervals always the same and, if not, when and in what way do they change? How are instruments adjusted to create the desired pitches? Does performing a note require holding an unvarying pitch or varying it in certain ways? Does playing 'in tune' with others mean playing the same pitch or two pitches that create a specific tuning beat, or any number of pitches within a small range? Different music traditions have answered such questions in a variety of ways and musical acculturation includes internalizing the tuning preferences of familiar traditions. (*Catherine Schmidt-Jones*)

Tyson, Florence (1918–2001)

American pioneer of MT born in Brooklyn, Tyson took the profession into new directions in the areas of psychiatry and psychology. Her training in art at Brooklyn College, coupled with an early career in advertising and fundraising led to her passion for the arts as an effective tool for many conditions. She established the first community-based MT organization in the USA in 1963, the Creative Arts Rehabilitation Center in New York and directed it until 1990. The Center was 'one of the first outpatient clinics in the United States to use music, dance, drama, painting, and poetry as therapy' (Saxon, 2001). Tyson was on the cutting edge of psychoanalytical MT, advocating for a continuum of care as well as through her grassroots emphasis on community mental health. She used case studies to convey the message and meaning of clinical work (Hadley, 2005). After her death, the Florence Tyson Fund was created to advance her vision (http://www.tysonfund.org). Her legacy is documented in McGuire (2004). (*Kevin Kirkland*)

U-based music therapy method

A receptive method mainly used in acute and chronic pain settings, based on the work in the 1970s of Jacques Jost, Jean-Marie Guiraud-Caladou ('U-shaped sequence') and validated by music therapist Dr Stéphane Guétin in many clinical studies (Guétin *et al.*, 2005). It assembles several pieces a few minutes each in length, melded and chained together to induce the client to gradually relax. The first effect is a decrease of musical rhythm, orchestration/instrumentation levels, frequency and volume (downward phase of the 'U'). The client then passes through the phase of maximum relaxation on the lower part of the 'U', which is then followed by a phase of re-dynamics (loudening) on the ascending right limb of the 'U'. Its effect, construction and application are comparable to a relaxation session or hypno-analgesia: the U-based musical sequence, 20–25 minutes long, is chosen by the client, based on their musical tastes, and is listened to on headphones in a quiet room (Jourt Pineau, 2012). (*Cécilia Jourt Pineau*)

unconditional positive regard

From humanistic psychology (Rogers), the therapist creates a safe, supportive space for positive change to take place by developing a caring and non-judgemental relationship with the client. It is an attitude of acceptance and liking toward the client to create a useful therapeutic relationship. By acceptance, we mean a warm regard of unconditional self-worth, of value no matter what the illness, condition, behaviour or feelings. It conveys a respect and a willingness to allow the client to possess their feelings their way. Rogers (1961) described it as a means of acceptance and regard for presenting attitudes, no matter how negative or positive, and no matter how much they may contradict other attitudes held in the past. 'This acceptance of each fluctuating aspect of this other person makes possible a relationship of warmth and safety, and the safety of being liked and prized as a person seems a highly important element in a helping profession' (Rogers, 1954). A similar term used by Heslop (1992) is 'non-possessive warmth'. (*Robin Rio*)

unconscious

Often mistakenly thought of as solely a warehouse of repressed memories or a zone of unawareness where one lacks insight into one's behaviours, scripts and actions. Jung, however, regarded the unconscious as a 'redeeming power of intelligence, creativity, and spiritual transcendence' (Fitzgerald, 1998: 269). Bruscia (in Karkou and Sanderson, 2006) used Priestley's analytic MT method to explore conscious or unconscious blocks through improvisation by identifying and entitling an issue for expression and investigation. Alfred Nieman (cited in Darnley-Smith and Patey, 2003) saw a link to the unconscious through the expression of emotion in sound (p. 4). Music seems to have the ability to bypass conscious rules and censorship, perhaps through processing abilities that access the unconscious more readily: 'Music therapy is appropriate for all patients regardless of their functional and cognitive levels because music has the power to provoke responses in us from both our conscious and our unconscious levels' (Tomaino, 2009: 212). Gardstrom (2008) would refer to this as music psychotherapy, where unconscious, often painful material is uncovered through the use of vocal and instrumental improvisation (pp. 149–500. See also the methods of Austin, 1999; Montello, 1998; Scheiby, 1998; or GIM: Bonny, 1975; Bruscia and Grocke, 2002). (*Kevin Kirkland*)

unichord tuning method

A non-traditional guitar technique in which the guitar is tuned to an open chord for the purpose of enabling certain clients to play the guitar (Cassity, 1977). The original tuning, recommended for nylon-string guitars, was an E-based tuning with the first string tuned to E^1 (first E above middle C), the second to B^{-1} (first

B below middle C), the third to $G\sharp^{-1}$, the fourth to E^{-1}, the fifth to B^{-2} and the sixth to E^{-2}. Cassity later recommended that guitars with steel or steel-blend strings use a D-based tuning, using the same ratios as the E-based tuning, to prevent the breaking of strings. Unichord tuning method may be used to play three-chord songs. The I chord is played by strumming the chord to which the guitar is tuned, the IV chord is played by barring all strings at the fifth fret and the V chord is played by barring all strings at the seventh fret. This method was successfully used with short-term adult psychiatric clients (Cassity, 1976) and with clients diagnosed with mild mental restriction (Cassity, 1977). (*Michael Cassity*)

validation

American social worker Naomi Feil created her Validation© approach (https://vfvalidation.org) between 1963 and 1980 as a more humanistic alternative to the traditional ways of working with older adults with dementia in care, whom she called the 'disoriented old-old' (Feil and de Klerk-Rubin, 1982: 9). Her approach and methods are now widely recognized and used by professionals throughout the world to help the older person with dementia tie up loose ends before dying, freely express feelings to resolve them and be validated for what she called 'intuitive wisdom' (Feil and de Klerk-Rubin, 1982: 44; Feil, 2002). Music therapists are also trained to meet and match the client – to 'walk by the person's side', adjusting and meeting the client in their gait, breathing and speech. Validation-trained therapists meet clients in their own memory and time, allowing them to feel heard and seen and, ultimately, to die with dignity and in peace. Feil is the author of two books, nine award-winning films and has gained international recognition for her groundbreaking work. (*Susan Summers*)

verbal counselling

This talk-based process uses an interpersonal professional relationship to facilitate individual change, development and self-awareness. Within this type of framework, the counsellor helps the client to work towards living both a resourceful and satisfying life. The counsellor also demonstrates full respect for each client and their right to self-determination. Individuals, couples, families and small groups may participate in and benefit from the work of counselling. Verbal counselling can focus on various things, such as coping with crises, communication challenges, relationship difficulties, action planning, resource identifying, decision making, emotional processing and skill building. The focus of each session depends on many factors, such as the client's goals and current state, their potential and motivation for change, the counsellor's level of training and experience and the overarching philosophy (Shebib, 2003). While MT is often viewed or defined as a nonverbal process, verbal counselling can be a key component to processing what arises through responses, relationships and interactions with music and the MT. (*Andrea Cave*)

Verdeau-Paillès psychomusical personality assessment (le bilan psycho-musical)

Developed by Jacqueline Verdeau-Paillès, French psychiatrist and *mt* who evaluated the interests and psychosocial states of MT clients. The 'bilan psycho-musical' assessment is divided into three stages: 1) a preliminary interview provides 'history of music and sound' of the client by engaging them to talk about their musical experiences, history, and personal and familial music; 2) a responsive test is based on the hearing ten extracts and sounds of varied according to a specific order of ten types of music: descriptive; heavy and anxious; emotional and sentimental; intimate and warm; surprising; calming; disconcerting; calming; Middle Eastern; stable and majestic. After each music selection the client is asked to freely express feelings and ideas verbally or through another expressive medium. The *mt* notes the responses, observes behaviour during testing, then groups them together as a table according to three broad groups of items to identify the receptive and communicative profile of the client; 3) during an active test, the *mt* observes and evaluates the spontaneous responses and behaviour of the client, who engages a small selection of instruments. (*Cécilia Jourt Pineau*)

vibration

Normally defined as mechanical oscillations with regards to a balance point, such as a swinging pendulum. The oscillations may be periodic or random. For instance, when an object such as a guitar is played, vibration occurs. The vibration is transmitted into the surrounding particles generating an acoustic wave which is transformed into sound by the human ear (López, 1970). Sound therapy is based on analyzing the impact of vibration on the human being. The acoustic energy of several instruments (Tibetan bowls, tuning forks, crystal quartz bowls, didgeridoo and even the human voice) also have an impact on the human body. Since the vibrations reach all the components of the human body, they could potentially contribute to the recovery of homeostatic balance. Sound therapy can be helpful when used as a relaxation procedure in order to decrease pain from both physical and mental diseases (Jauset, 2011). (*Jordi A. Jauset*)

vibroacoustic therapy

An approach to low frequency sound therapy developed by Olav Skille (1997) in Norway between 1968 and 1980. It was first applied to developmentally delayed children with a prototype in 1980. It uses sinusoidal sound of 30–120 Hz, with particular emphasis on 40 Hz, 52 Hz, 68 Hz and 86 Hz. Treatment involves application of a single frequency that is modulated with a steady rise and fall of amplitude at a rate of about six to eight seconds from peak to peak. A noteworthy application of this method in research was done by Wigram (1996). (*Lee Bartel*)

visual cortex

Processes visual information and is located in the occipital lobe. It receives visual information from the retina via relay through the lateral geniculate nuclei and is topographically represented such that the each side of the brain receives information exclusively from that contralateral hemivisual field. The area adjacent to the dominant (usually left side) visual cortex and the parietal and temporal cortices is involved in language processing, such as reading and comprehension of language. Platel and Baron found that Brodmann's area 18 and 19 in the visual cortex may create an image/symbol in this 'mind's eye' region to help to decipher changes in pitch (Platel, 2005). The visual cortex is also activated when reading or imagining a score (Fick and Shilts, 2006). (*Robin Hsiung and Kevin Kirkland*)

vitality affects (dynamics)

Emotions differ in intensity and duration. For decades, the developmental psychologist Daniel Stern has studied specific and often neglected type of emotions with low intensity and short duration. 'Many qualities of feeling that occur do not fit into our existing lexicon or taxonomy of affects. These elusive qualities are better captured by dynamic, kinetic terms, such as "surging", "fading away", "fleeting", "explosive", "crescendo", "decrescendo", "bursting", "drawn out", and so on' (Stern 1985a: 54). Stern has used different concepts, including 'vitality affects', to describe these dynamic forms that permeate everyday life, psychology, psychotherapy and the arts. Vitality dynamics have five specific and theoretically different elements: movement, time, force, space and intention/directionality, and can be studied through microanalysis (Stern, 2010). Such dynamic forms of vitality are identifiable in sounds and corporeal and facial movements in neonate and infant MT. The experience of vitality is characterized as what Stern (1985a) calls 'vitality affects' such as a sense of sudden explosiveness and fleetingness. Stern claims that infants experience vitality affects more directly than adults. Smeijsters' theory of analogy refers to the concept of 'vitality affects'. Pavlicevic (1997) refers to Stern in her overview of the music and meaning debate, including the presentation of her own influential concept of 'dynamic form'. (*Lars Ole Bonde and Jin Hyun Kim*)

vocables

Sung syllables with no textual meaning. They are used in a wide variety of music styles, such as yodelling traditions, jazz scat singing and pop-music beat-boxing. Using vocables allows the singer to choose a syllable for aesthetic reasons, such as the timbre of a vowel sound or percussive quality of a consonant and obviates the need for a suitable text. As with instrumental music, emotions and meaning are expressed nonverbally, through musical elements such as melody, rhythm and dynamics. (*Catherine Schmidt-Jones*)

vocal holding stages

Vocal holding techniques are not meant to be prescriptive and are not necessarily used in the order that follows but, for the sake of clarity, the process is described as it complements the developmental stages that may have to be re-experienced to provide a reparative experience for the client (Austin, 2009). In the initial vocal holding phase, the client and the *mt* sing in unison, providing an environment in which the client can re-experience a symbiotic way of being. Harmonizing creates the opportunity for the client to experience a sense of being separate yet in relationship. Mirroring occurs when the client sings a melodic line and the therapist responds by repeating the client's melody back to them, thus providing an experience of being heard and validated. Grounding occurs when the therapist sings the tone or root of the chords and the client can improvise freely and return to the grounding tone when and if more support is needed; a musical intervention that is reminiscent of a typical pattern of interaction between the child and the maternal figure that occurs when the child begins to move away from the mother or primary caregiver to explore the environment (rapprochement). (*Diane Austin*)

vocal holding techniques

These are integral to vocal psychotherapy. Defined by Austin (2009), they involve the intentional use of two alternating chords in combination with the therapist's voice to create a consistent and stable musical environment that facilitates improvised singing within the client therapist relationship. This improvisational structure is limited to two chords to establish a predictable, secure, musical and psychological container that will enable clients to relinquish some of the mind's control, sink down into their bodies and allow their spontaneous selves to emerge in the music. The simplicity of the music and the hypnotic and trustworthy repetition of the two chords, combined with the rocking rhythmic motion and the singing of single syllables (sounds, not words initially) by both client and therapist, can produce an altered state and easier access to the unconscious. (*Diane Austin*)

vocal learning

Researchers Patel and Iversen (Strickland, 2011) have found that humans process the ability to step to the beat through the intertwining of the hearing system with the motor control systems. They say that this connection has allowed humans to learn to speak. Called a vocal learning brain, humans are one of a very small number of species (parrots and dolphins are other examples) that can follow the beat – sometimes referred to as the seventh sense – which points to the concept of rhythm and the ability to follow it, as a foundation of language. A team of Mexican researchers attempted to train monkeys to tap to the beat of a metronome. They could respond after the beat but never with it, which is an important distinction between any brain's ability to learn, anticipate or simply respond to a stimulus (Patel, 2008). The vocal learning hypothesis is seen as a tightly integrated sound and movement: a vocal-learning brain involves the basal ganglia to move to the beat. The basal ganglia are connected to auditory regions. (*Kevin Kirkland*)

vocal psychotherapy

Vocal psychotherapy is a new model of music psychotherapy developed by Diane Austin (2009). It is defined as the use of the breath, sound, vocal improvisation, songs and dialogue within a client–therapist relationship to promote intra-psychic and interpersonal growth and change. In vocal psychotherapy, there is an organic flow between music and words; the words take the music to a deeper level and the music takes the words to a deeper level. Since the *mt* is working with unconscious contents, including regression in service of the self, re-enactments, dissociation and other symptoms of trauma, advanced training is necessary. Although originally used with individual adults, vocal psychotherapy has also been adapted for work with many diverse populations and groups. (*Diane Austin*)

vocal therapy

A specialized treatment and training system based on the principles and main rules of classical singing (bel canto) developed by Shushardzhan (1994). The method involves an effective system of voice training studies, after which the voice is used as the tool of treatment in health protection and strengthening. Specific exercises stimulate vocal vibrations, especially the cardiovascular and respiratory systems. Positive outcomes are suggested in the treatment of bronchial asthma and chronic bronchitis, cardiovascular pathology, neurosis and speech disorders (Shushardzhan, 1995, 1999). It is theorized that vocal therapy activates preserved and intellectual–creative abilities of the client. (*Sergey Shushardzhan*)

voice

The sound produced in the larynx by the vibration of the vocal cords (also called folds). Speaking and singing involve a voice mechanism that is composed of three subsystems: air pressure system, vibratory system and resonating system. Through two basic categories of meaningful sounds, vowels and consonants, the voice conveys information about the speaking individual (Fogerty and Kewley-Port, 2008). MT methods that primarily use voice can include vocal improvisation, singing, toning, chanting, vocal psychotherapy and melodic intonation therapy. (*Ivana Ilic*)

voice movement therapy

A particular approach to therapeutic voice work developed by Paul Newham (1999) for those whose expressive capacity has been detrimentally impacted by emotional issues, trauma, neurodegenerative disease, physical ailment and mental illness. Voice movement therapy is useful for clients with history of not asserting or expressing themselves. It also applies to those whose social or professional predicament places exceptional demands upon the voice and where clients can benefit from education and rehabilitation in the care of their voice. For others, the potential for expression and creativity through singing and sound making is central to the method (Newham, 1999: 15–16). (*Kevin Kirkland*)

whistling

Most people remember the famous whistling chorus of the *Colonel Bogey March* during the 1957 movie *Bridge over the River Kwai* when the prisoners of war enter the camp. Whistling has been uses for centuries to occupy the mind on positive mood states, even during mundane tasks, as well as part of celebrations in African and Celtic societies. It is only in the past century or two that whistling became, in the West, an activity associated with males while being decidedly unladylike for a woman to whistle. As one elderly woman once quoted (personal communication, 2011), 'A whistling woman and a crowing hen are neither fit for God nor men'. This often neglected ancient skill can be incorporated into MT as an alternate form of personal vocal expression, for music games, and more. (*Kevin Kirkland*)

whole-tone scale

A scale made up entirely of whole steps and containing only six notes within an octave. There are only two forms of the whole-tone scale: the first form, containing the note C, is variously labelled WT I, WT A, or WT 0 (since 0 is the pitch-class label for the note C): C D E F♯ G♯ A♯. The second form, containing C♯/Db is labelled WT II, WT B, or WT 1: Db, Eb, F, G, A, B. While fragments of whole tone scales can be found in any era of tonal music, it first came to be used in its own right during the late nineteenth and twentieth centuries by composers such as Debussy, Bartok, Stravinsky, Crumb and Messiaen. Because these scales lack half steps and perfect fifths, normal tonal relationships are impossible. They have often been used where tonal vagueness, a sense of exploration or a suggestion of the supernatural is desired. (*Peter Martens*)

Wigram, Tony (1953–2011)

Internationally renowned British-Danish *mt*, researcher, educator and mentor. Born in London, UK, Wigram studied music at Bristol University and MT under Juliette Alvin at the Guildhall School of Music and Drama, qualifying in 1975. In

1992, he became professor of MT at Aalborg University in Denmark, while still researching and living in the UK with his violinist wife Jenny and their three sons. Appointed Head of PhD studies at Aalborg in 1997, he nurtured a new generation of researchers. Wigram's clinical research was centred on MT in distinguishing autism spectrum disorders from other communication disabilities, with interests in Rett's syndrome, vibroacoustic MT, assessment and teaching improvisation. He wrote or edited 14 books, over 50 articles and over 70 chapters. As a world leader, Wigram was President of the European MT Confederation (1994–1998), President of the WFMT (1996–99), Professor of MT at Anglia Ruskin University and Honorary Principal Research Fellow in the Faculty of Music, University of Melbourne. His major publications are listed in the references. (*Jenny Wigram, Felicity Baker and Lars Ole Bonde*)

womb sounds

The fetus receives rich and diverse information through sound. The pregnant mother's body is not silent, so the baby's aural environment is made up of a constant, stimulating and very complex sound universe (Federico and Whitwell, 2001). Some of the sounds are working constantly (the mother's heartbeat, blood circulation and breathing movements), while others are less regular sounds such as those made by internal fluids, muscular movements and the mother's voice. The noises which form the intrauterine sound environment range approximately between 70 dB and 84 dB in intensity (Lecanuet, 1996). By the end of the pregnancy, the baby's hearing system is able to perceive the mother's intestinal noises as low as 60 dB (Spence and DeCasper, 1987; Abrams *et al.*, 1998). The fetus requires all this auditory stimulation, which contributes to the development of their nervous system. The baby's hearing system is fully developed approximately three and a half months into the pregnancy. Only then is the baby capable of perceiving, first the intrauterine sounds (between the tenth and twelfth week) (Hepper and Shahidullah, 1994) and, later, from the fourth month on, the sounds from the outside world which begin to filter inside (sixteenth week) (Birnholz and Benacellaf, 1983; Crade and Lovett, 1988; Federico and Whitwell, 2001). This does not, however, mean that their brains are capable of decoding all this information. Babies are continuously developing but, during the fourth month, many functions are still too immature. (*Gabriel Federico*)

Yamamatsu method

Influenced by Juliet Alvin's visits to Japan, Tadafumi Yamamatsu developed the use of Roger's client-centred therapy and Altshuler's (1948) ISO principle by matching the client's mood then engaging in client–therapist improvisation and interaction for here-and-now communication. His method emphasizes the therapist's sensitive responses and flexibility while emphasizing the client's positive and healthy components (Haneishi, 2005: 266–267). (*Kevin Kirkland*)

References

Abrams, B. (2005) Evaluating qualitative music therapy research. In B. L. Wheeler (ed.) *Music Therapy Research*, 2nd edn. Gilsum, NH: Barcelona Publishers, pp. 246–58.

Abrams, B. (2010) Evidence-based music therapy practice: An integral understanding. *Journal of Music Therapy*, 47(3), 351–79.

Abrams, B. (2011) Understanding music as a temporal–aesthetic way of being: implications for a general theory of music therapy. *Arts in Psychotherapy*, 38(2), 114–19.

Abrams, B. and Meadows, T. (2005) Personal construct psychology and the repertory grid technique. In B. Wheeler (ed.) *Music Therapy Research*, 2nd edn. Gilsum, NH: Barcelona Publishers, pp. 472–86.

Abrams, R. M., Griffiths, S. K., Wang, X., Sain, J., Langford, G. and Gerhardt, K. J. (1998) Fetal music perception: The role of sound transmission. *Music Perception*, 15, 307–17.

Abukishek, I. F. (2011) *Human Rights and Democracy in Palestine: Their value for the new generation.* (Doctoral dissertation, Northeastern University). Retrieved from IRis Law and Public Policy Dissertations. Paper 3. http://hdl.handle.net/2047/d200002046

Ackerman, D. (1990) *A Natural History of the Senses*. New York: Random House.

Agency for Healthcare Research and Quality (2009) Evidence based practice. Retrieved from http://effectivehealthcare.ahrq.gov/

Agrotou, A. (1998) Psychodynamic group music therapy with profoundly learning disabled residents and their carers. Developing a theory and practice for the realisation of therapeutic aims for residents and the acquirement of therapist's skills by carers. (Unpublished doctoral dissertation). University of Sheffield, Sheffield, UK.

Ahessy, B. (2011) Lesbian, gay and bisexual issues in music therapy training and education: The love that dares not sing its name. *Canadian Journal of Music Therapy*, 17(1), 11–33.

Ahonen-Eerikäinen, H. (1999) *Samalle Aaltopituudelle*. Helsinki: Kirjayhtymä Oy.

Ahonen-Eerikäinen, H. (2007) *Group Analytic Music Therapy*. Gilsum, NH: Barcelona Publishers.

Aigen, K. (1991) *The Roots of Music Therapy: Towards an indigenous research paradigm.* (Doctoral dissertation, New York University). Available from Dissertation Abstracts International, 52(6), 1933A UMI Dissertation Publishing, Order 9134717.

Aigen, K. (2005a) *Music-centered Music Therapy*. Gilsum, NH: Barcelona Publishers.

Aigen, K. (2005b) *Being in Music: Foundations of Nordoff–Robbins music therapy*. Gilsum, NH: Barcelona Publishers.

Aigen, K. (2005c) *Playing in the Band: A qualitative study of popular music styles as clinical improvisation*. Gilsum, NH: Barcelona Publishing.

Aigen, K. (2008) An analysis of qualitative music therapy research reports 1987–2006: Articles and book chapters. *The Arts in Psychotherapy*, 35, 251–61.

Aigen, K., Miller, C. K., Kim, Y., Pasiali, V., Kwak, E.-M. and Tague, D. B. (2007) Nordoff–Robbins Music Therapy. In A.-A. Darrow (ed.) *Introduction to approaches in music therapy*. Silver Spring, MD: AMTA, pp. 63–77.

Aldridge, D. (1996) *From Out of the Silence: Music therapy research and practice in medicine*. London: Jessica Kingsley Publishers.

Aldridge, D. (1999) *Suicide: The tragedy of hopelessness*. London: Jessica Kingsley.

Aldridge, D. (2003) Music therapy and spirituality: A transcendental understanding of suffering. Music Therapy Today (online) February, http://www.musictherapyworld.net

Aldridge, D. (2005a) *Case Study Designs in Music Therapy*. London: Jessica Kingsley.

Aldridge, G. (2005b) Therapeutic narrative analysis as a narrative case study approach. In D. Aldridge (ed.) *Case Study Designs in Music Therapy*. London: Jessica Kingsley, pp. 31–52.

Aldridge, D. (2006) Music therapy and spirituality: A transcendental understanding of suffering. In D. Aldridge and J. Facher (eds) *Music and Altered States: Consciousness, transcendence, therapy, and addictions*. London: Jessica Kingsley, pp. 172–83.

Aldridge, G. and Aldridge, D. (2008) *Melody in Music Therapy: A therapeutic narrative analysis*. London: Jessica Kingsley.

Aldridge, D. and Facher, J. (eds) (2006) *Music and Altered States: Consciousness, transcendence, therapy, and addictions*. London: Jessica Kingsley.

Allen-Meares, P. and Fraser, M. (2004) *Interventions with Children and Adolescents: An interdisciplinary perspective*. Boston, MA: Pearson Education.

Altshuler, I. M. (1943) Four year's experience with music as a therapeutic agent at Eloise Hospital, Michigan Detroit. *American Journal of Psychiatry*, 100, 792–4.

Altshuler, I. M. (1945) The organism as a whole and music therapy. *Sociometry*, 8(3–4), 227–32.

Altshuler, I. M. (1948) A psychiatrist's experiences with music as a therapeutic agent. In D. Schullian and M. Schoen (eds) *Music and Medicine*. New York: Henry Schuman, pp. 266–81.

Altshuler, I. M. (1952) *Music Therapy: Retrospect and perspective*. Lawrence, KS: Allen Press.

Alvesson, M. and Sköldberg, K. (2009) *Reflexive Methodology: New vistas for qualitative research*, 2nd edn. London: Sage Publishers.

Alvin, J. (1965/1978) *Music for the Handicapped Child*. London: Oxford University Press.

Alvin, J. (1966) *Music Therapy*. New York: Basic Books.

Alvin, J. (1975) *Music Therapy*, rev. edn. London: Hutchinson.

Alvin, J. and Warwick, A. (1991) *Music Therapy for the Autistic Child*, 2nd edn. Oxford: Oxford University Press.

American Orff-Schulwerk Association (2013) What is Orff-Schulwerk? Retrieved from http://www.aosa.org/orff.html

Amir, D. (2005) Grounded theory. In B. L. Wheeler (ed.) *Music Therapy Research*, 2nd edn. Gilsum, NH: Barcelona Publishers, pp. 365–78.

Amnesty International (2011) *Learn about Human Rights*. Amnesty International. Retrieved from http://amnesty.org/en/human-rights

AMTA (2009) Professional competencies. American Music Therapy Association. Retrieved from http://www.musictherapy.org/about/competencies/

AMTA (2010) *Definition of Evidence-based Music Therapy*. Paper presented at the

Practice adopted by the Board of the American Music Therapy Association, Cleveland, OH.

AMTA (2011) What is music therapy? American Music Therapy Association. Retrieved from http://www.musictherapy.org/about/musictherapy/

Anderson, C. L., Krebaum, S. R. (1998) *An Analysis of the Psychiatric Music Questionnaire (PMTQ) and Standard Personality Questionnaires*. Paper presented at the AMTA Annual Conference, Cleveland, OH.

Andreasen, N. C. and Black, D. W. (eds) (1995) *Introductory Textbook of Psychiatry*, 2nd edn. Washington, DC: American Psychiatric Press.

Ansdell, G. (1996) Talking about music therapy: A dilemma and a qualitative experiment. *British Journal of Music Therapy*, 19(1): 4-15.

Ansdell, G. (2006) [Review of] Music as therapy: A dialogical perspective by Rudy Garred. *British Journal of Music Therapy*, 20(2): 133.

Ansdell, G. (2010a) Belonging through musicking: Explorations of musical community. In B. Stige, G. Ansdell, C. Elefant and M. Pavlicevic (eds) *Where Music Helps*. Aldershot: Ashgate Publishing Ltd, pp. 41–62.

Ansdell, G. (2010b) Where performing helps: Processes and affordances of performance in community music therapy. In B. Stige, G. Ansdell, C. Elefant and M. Pavlicevic (eds) *Where Music Helps: Community music therapy in action and reflection*. Aldershot: Ashgate Publishing, pp. 161–86.

Ashida, S. (2000) The effect of reminiscence music therapy sessions on changes in depressive symptoms in elderly persons with dementia. *Journal of Music Therapy*, 37(3), 170–82.

Association for Music and Imagery (2011) The Bonny Method. Association for Music and Imagery. Retrieved from http://www.ami-bonnymethod.org/the-bonny-method-2/

Auf der Heide, T. M. C. (2012) *Interpersonal rhythms disrupted by a history of trauma: An in-depth case study of analytical music therapy*. Unpublished Dissertation. Columbia City University, NY:

Austin, D. (1999) Vocal improvisation in analytically oriented music therapy with adults. In T. Wigram and J. De Backer (eds) *Clinical Applications of Music Therapy in Psychiatry*. London: Jessica Kingsley, pp. 141–57.

Austin, D. (2009) *The Theory and Practice of Vocal Psychotherapy: Songs of the self*. London: Jessica Kingsley.

Austin, D. and Dvorkin, J. M. (1993) Resistance in individual music therapy. *The Arts in Psychotherapy*, 20(5), 423–9.

Ayers, A. J. (1961) Development of body scheme for children. *American Journal of Occupational Therapy*, 15, 99–102.

Ayers, J. (1979) *Sensory Integration and the Child*. Los Angeles, CA: Western Psychological Services.

Badia, L. M. (2001) *Music and Trance*. (Unpublished doctoral dissertation). Carlos Albizu University, Miami, FL.

Baines, D. (2011) *Doing Anti-oppressive Practice: Social justice social work*. Halifax, NS: Fernwood Publishing.

Baines, S. (1992a) A consumer-directed and partnered community mental health music therapy program: program development and evaluation. *Canadian Journal of Music Therapy*, 7(1), 51–70.

Baines, S. (1992b) *A Sociocultural and Political Analysis of Music Therapy: A question of ethics*. (Unpublished masters thesis). New York University, New York.

Baines, S. and Danko, G. (2010) Community music therapy in community mental health: A consumer initiated song-based paradigm. *Canadian Journal of Music Therapy*, 16(1), 148–91.

Baker, F. A. (2000) Modifying melodic intonation therapy programs for adults with severe non-fluent aphasia. *Music Therapy Perspectives*, 2, 107–11.

Baker, F. A. (2011) Facilitating neurological reorganization through music therapy: A case example of modified melodic intonation therapy in the treatment of a person with aphasia. In A. Meadows (ed.) *Developments in Music Therapy Practice: Case perspectives*. Gilsum, NH: Barcelona Publishers, pp. 281–97.

Baker, F. A., Gleadhill, L. M. and Dingle, G. A. (2007) Music therapy and emotional exploration: Exposing substance abuse clients to the experiences of non-drug induced emotions. *Arts in Psychotherapy*, 34, 321–30.

Baker, F. A. and Uhlig, S. (2011) Diversity in approaches to therapeutic voice work: Developing a model of voicework in music therapy. In F. A. Baker and S. Uhlig (eds) *Voicework in Music Therapy: Research and practice*. London Jessica Kingsley, pp. 333–50.

Baker, F. A., Wigram, T., Stott, D. and McFerran, K. (2008) Therapeutic songwriting in music therapy: Part 1. Who are the therapists, who are the clients, and why is songwriting used? *Nordic Journal of Music Therapy*, 17, 105–23.

Baker, F. A., Wigram, T., Stott, D. and McFerran, K. (2009) Therapeutic songwriting in music therapy: Comparing the literature with practice across diverse populations. *Nordic Journal of Music Therapy*, 18, 32–56.

Baker, M. (2007) Music moves brain to pay attention, Stanford study finds. *Stanford School of Medicine News Releases*, 1 August. Retrieved from http://med.stanford.edu/news_releases/2007/july/music.html

Ball, P. (2010) *The Music Instinct: How much works and why we can't do without it.* Oxford: Oxford University Press.

Balzer, H. U. (2009) Chronobiology as a foundation for and an approach to a new understanding of the influence of music. In R. Haas and V. Brandes (eds) *Music that Works: Contributions of biology, neurophysiology, psychology, medicine, and musicology.* Vienna: Springer.

Bamberger, J. (2006) What develops in musical development? In G. E. McPherson (ed.) *The Child as Musician: A handbook of musical development.* Oxford: Oxford University Press, pp. 69–81.

Barbour, I. G. (1974) *Myths, Models, and Paradigms: A comparative study in science and religion.* New York: Harper & Row.

Barbour, R. (2001) Checklists for improving rigor in qualitative research: A case of the tail wagging the dog? *British Medical Journal*, 322, 1115–17.

Barbour, R. (2003) The newfound credibility of qualitative research? Tales of technical essentialism and co-option. *Qualitative Health Research*, 13(7), 1019–27.

Bar-Even, R. and Pridor, S. (2010) *Dynamic Batukada.* Paper presented at the World Music Therapy Congress, Cadiz, Spain.

Bargiel, M. (2004) Lullabies and play songs: Theoretical considerations for an early attachment music therapy intervention through parental singing for developmentally at-risk infants. *Voices: A World Forum for Music Therapy*, 4(1).

Barry, P., O'Callaghan, C., Wheeler, G. and Grocke, D. E. (2010) Music therapy CD creation for initial pediatric radiation therapy: A mixed methods analysis. *Journal of Music Therapy*, 47(3), 233–63.

Bear, M. F., Connors, B. W. and Paradiso, M. A. (2007) *Neuroscience: Exploring the brain*. Philadelphia, PA: Lippincott Williams & Wilkins.

Beck, U., Giddens, A. and Lash, S. (1994) *Reflexive Modernization: Politics, tradition, and aesthetics in the modern social order*. Cambridge: Polity Press.

Beebe, B. and Lachmann, F. (1994) Representations and internalizations on infancy: Three principles of salience. *Psychoanalytic Psychology*, 11(2), 127–65.

Benenzon, R. (1971) *Musicoterapia y Educación*. Buenos Aires: Ed. Paidós.

Benenzon, R. (1976) *Musicoterapia en la Psicosis Infatil*. Buenos Aires: Ed. Paidós.

Benenzon, R. (1985a) *Manual de Musicoterapia*. Barcelona: Ed. Paidós.

Benenzon, R. (1985b) Algunos pensamientos sobre el rol de la musicoterapia en el campo de la salud. *Orientación Musicoterapie*, 3(11).

Benenzon, R. (1988) *Teorio de Musicoterapia*. Sao Paulo: Summus.

Benenzon, R. (1997) *Music Therapy Theory and Manual: Contributions to the knowledge of nonverbal contexts*, 2nd edn. Springfield, IL: Charles C. Thomas.

Benenzon, R. (2000) *Music Therapy: From theory to practice*. Barcelona: Paidós.

Bengtsson, S. L. (2007) Cortical regions involved in the generation of musical structures during improvisation in pianists. *Journal of Cognitive Neuroscience*, 19(5), 830–42.

Berger, D. S. (2002) *Music Therapy, Sensory Integration, and the Autistic Child*. London: Jessica Kingsley.

Bergstrøm-Nielsen, C. (2010) Graphica notation: The simple sketch and beyond. *Nordic Journal of Music Therapy*, 19(2), 162–77.

Bernstein, N. (1967) *Coordination and Regulation of Movements*. New York: Pergamon.

Bion, W. R. (1962) *A Theory of Thinking: In second thoughts*. London: Karnac Books.

Bion, W. R. (1970) *Attention and Interpretation*. London: Karnac Books.

Birnholz, J. C. and Benacellaf, B. R. (1983) The development of the human fetal hearing. *Science*, 222, 516–18.

Bitcon, C. (2000) *Alike and Different: The clinical and educational uses of Orff-Schulwerk*, 2nd edn. New Braunfels, TX: Barcelona Publishers.

Bittman, B., Berk, L., Shannon, M., Sharaf, M., Westengard, J., Guegler, K. J. and Ruf, D. W. (2005) Recreational music-making modulates the human stress response: A preliminary individualized gene expression strategy. *Medical Science Monitor*, 11(2), 31–40.

Blood, A. J., Zatorre, R. J., Bermudez, P. and Evans, A. C. (1999) Emotional responses to pleasant and unpleasant music correlate with activity in paralimbic brain regions. *Nature Neuroscience*, 2(4), 382–7.

Blumenbach, J. F. (1779) *Handbuch der Naturgeschichte*. Göttingen: J. C. Dieterich.

Bohlmeijer, E., Roemer, M., Cuijpers, P. and Smit, F. (2007) The effect of reminiscence on psychological well-being in older adults: a meta-analysis. *Aging and Mental Health*, 11, 291–300.

Bohnert, K. (1999) Meaningful musical experience and the treatment of an individual in psychosis: a case study. *Music Therapy Perspectives*, 17, 69–73.

Bonde, L. O. (2000) Metaphor and narrative in Guided Imagery and Music. *Journal of the Association for Music Therapy*, 7, 59–76.

Bonde, L. O. (2005) *The Bonny Method of Guided Imagery and Music (BMGIM) with Cancer Survivors: A psychosocial study with focus on the influence of BMGIM on mood and quality of life*. (Unpublished doctoral dissertation). Aalborg University, Aalborg, Denmark.

Bonde, L. O. (2011) Health music(k)ing – music therapy or music and health? A model, empirical examples, and personal reflections. *Music and Arts in Action. Special Issue:*

Health promotion and wellness, 3(2), 120–40.
Bonde, L. O. (2013) Using mixed methods in music therapy health care research: Reflections on the relationship between research question, design, and methods in the research project Receptive music therapy with female cancer patients in rehabilitation. In G. S. Reinbacker (ed.) *I: Research design. Validation in social sciences*. Videnbasen: Aalborg Universitet.
Bonny, H. (1975) Music and consciousness. *Journal of Music Therapy*, 12(3), 121–35.
Bonny, H. (1978/2002) *GIM Monograph #2: The role of tape music programs in the GIM process*. Salina, KS: Bonny Foundation.
Bonny, H. (1998) *Basic Premises of GIM Guided Imagery and Music: The Bonny Method and beyond*. Gilsum, NH: Barcelona.
Bonny, H. (1999a) *Five International Models of Music Therapy*. Paper presented at the World Congress of Music Therapy, Washington, DC.
Bonny, H. (1999b) Music and consciousness. *Nordic Journal of Music Therapy*, 8(2), 171–9.
Bonny, H. (2002) *Music and Consciousness: The evolution of guided imagery and music*. Edited by Lisa Summer. Gilsum, NH: Barcelona Publishers.
Booth, P. B. and Jernberg, A. M. (2010) *Theraplay: Helping parents and children build better relationships through attachment-based play*. San Francisco, CA: Wiley.
Borczon, R. M. (1997) *Music Therapy: Group vignettes*. Gilsum, NH: Barcelona Publishers.
Bordin, E. S. (1979) The generalizability of the psychoanalytic concept of the working alliance. *Psychotherapy: Theory, Research and Practice*, 16(3), 252–60.
Bowen, C. M., Yates, G. N. and Palmer, S. (2010) *A Relationship Approach to Rehabilitation: Thinking about relationships after brain injury*. London: Karnac Publishers.
Bower, J. and Shoemark, H. (2009) Music therapy to promote interpersonal interactions in early paediatric neurorehabilitation. *Australian Journal of Music Therapy*, 20, 59–75.
Boxill, E. (1981) A continuum of awareness: Music therapy with the developmentally handicapped. *Music Therapy*, 1(1), 17–23.
Boxill, E. (1997a) *The miracle of music therapy*. Gilsum, NH: Barcelona Publishers.
Boxill, E. (1997b) *Students Against Violence Everywhere – S.A.V.E. – Through Music Therapy: A manual of guidelines, music therapy interventions, music activities, music materials*. New York: Music Therapists for Peace, Inc.
Boxill, E. H. (1985) *Music Therapy for the Developmentally Disabled*. Rockville, MD: Aspen.
Boxill, E. H. (1988) Continuing notes: Worldwide networking for peace. *Music Therapy*, 7(1), 80–1.
Boxill, E. H. (1991) *La Musicoterapia per Babini Disabili*. Turin, Italy: Omega.
Boyd, R. and Myers, J. (1988) Transformative education. *International Journal of Lifelong Education*, 7(4), 261–84.
Bradley, S. (2000) *Affect Regulation and the Development of Psychopathology*. New York: Guildford Press.
Braswell, C. H., Buttram, J. B., Goldstein, H. K., Ott, W. H. and Schoenberger, L. (1970) The influence of music therapy on vocational potential. *Journal of Music Therapy*, 7, 28–38.
Bregman, A. (1990) *Auditory Scene Analysis: The perceptual organisation of sound*. Cambridge, MA: MIT Press.
Briggs, C. (1991) A model for understanding musical development. *Music Therapy*, 10(1), 1–21.

Bronfenbrenner, U. (1979) *The Ecology of Human Development: Experiments by nature and design*. Cambridge, MA: Harvard University Press.

Broucek, M. (1987) Beyond healing to 'whole-ing': a voice for the deinstitutionalization of music therapy. *Music Therapy*, 6(2), 50–8.

Brown, S. (2000) The 'musilanguage' model of human evolution. In N. L. Wallin, B. Merker and S. Brown (eds) *The Origins of Music*. Cambridge, MA: Massachusetts Institute of Technology, pp. 271–300.

Brown, S., Martinez, M. J. and Parsons, L. M. (2006) Music and language side by side in the brain: A PET study of the generation of melodies and sentences. *European Journal of Neurosciences*, 23, 2791–803.

Brown, T. and Kozak, A. (1998) Emotion and the possibility of psychologists entering into heaven. In M. F. Mascolo and S. Griffin (eds) *What Develops in Emotional Development?* New York: Plenum, pp. 135–55.

Bruer, R. A., Spitznagel, E. and Cloninger, C. R. (2007) The temporal limits of cognitive changes from music therapy in elderly persons with dementia or dementia-like cognitive impairment: A randomized controlled trial. *Music Therapy*, 44(4), 308–28.

Bruscia, K. E. (1987a) Sixty-four clinical techniques. In K. E. Bruscia (ed.) *Improvisational Models of Music Therapy*. Springfield, IL: Charles C. Thomas, pp. 536–57.

Bruscia, K. E. (1987b) *Improvisational Models of Music Therapy*. Springfield, IL: Charles C. Thomas.

Bruscia, K. E. (1991) *Case Studies in Music Therapy*. Gilsum, NH: Barcelona Publishers.

Bruscia, K. E. (1995) Modes of consciousness in Guided Imagery and Music (GIM): A therapist's experience of the guiding process. In C. Kenny (ed.) *Listening, Playing, Creating: Essays on the power of sound*. Albany, NY: State University of New York Press.

Bruscia, K. E. (1998a) Techniques for uncovering and working with countertransference. In K. E. Bruscia (ed.) *The Dynamics of Music Psychotherapy*. Gilsum, NH: Barcelona Publishers, pp. 93–116.

Bruscia, K. E. (1998b) *Defining Music Therapy*, 2nd edn. Gilsum, NH: Barcelona Publishers.

Bruscia, K. E. (1998c) Standards of integrity for qualitative music therapy research. *Journal of Music Therapy*, 35(3), 176–200.

Bruscia, K. E. (1998d) Manifestations of transference in Guided Imagery and Music. In K. Bruscia (ed.) *The Dynamics of Music Psychotherapy*. Gilsum, NH: Barcelona Publishers, pp. 407–30.

Bruscia, K. E. (1998e) An introduction to music psychotherapy In K. E. Bruscia (ed.) *The dynamics of music psychotherapy*. Gilsum, NH: Barcelona Publishers, pp. 1–16.

Bruscia, K. E. (2002) Foreword. In Stige, B. *Culture-Centered Music Therapy*. Gilsum, NH: Barcelona Publishers.

Bruscia, K. E. (2005) First person research. In B. Wheeler (ed.) *Music Therapy Research*, 2nd edn. Gilsum, NH: Barcelona Publishers.

Bruscia, K. E. and Grocke, D. E. (eds) (2002) *Guided Imagery and Music: The Bonny Method and beyond*. Gilsum, NH: Barcelona Publishers.

Buber, M. (1958) *I and Thou*, 2nd edn. (translated by R. G. Smith). New York: Charles Scribner's Sons.

Bunt, L. (1994) *Music Therapy: An art beyond words*. London: Routledge.

Bunt, L. (2004) Mary Priestley interviewed by Leslie Bunt. *Voices: A world forum for music therapy*, 4(2). Retrieved from https://normt.uib.no/index.php/voices/article/viewArticle/180/139

Bunt, L. and Hoskyns, S. (2002) *The Handbook of Music Therapy*. East Sussex: Brunner-Routledge.

Bush, D., Clark, M., Clarkson, G., Goldberg, F., Lewis, K., Mardis, L., Merritt, S., Stokes-Stearns, S. (2002) The fundamentals of the Bonny Method. In K. E. Bruscia and D. E. Grocke (eds) *Guided Imagery and Music: The Bonny method and beyond*. Gilsum, NH: Barcelona Publishers.

Cadrin, M. L. (2006) Music therapy legacy work in palliative care: Creating meaning at end of life. *Canadian Journal of Music Therapy*, 12(1), 109–37.

Campbell, J. (1973) *Myths to Live By*. New York: Bantam Books.

Campbell, J. and Moyers, B. (1988) *The Power of Myth*. New York: Doubleday.

Campbell, R. (1989) *Psychiatric Dictionary*. New York: Oxford University Press.

CAMT (1994) Music therapy. Annual General Meeting of the Canadian Association for Music Therapy, Vancouver, British Columbia, Canada.

Carlsson, T. (2007) *Varhainen Vuorovaikutus ja Musiikkiterapia*. Open University of the University of Jyväskylän, Jyväskylä, Finland.

Carmichael, D. (2011/12) Collaborative health care. *Canadian Health and Lifestyle*, Winter, 30–2.

Carpente, J. (2011) Addressing core features of autism: Integrating Nordoff–Robbins music therapy within the developmental, individual difference, relationship-based-DIR floortime model. In A. Meadows (ed.) *Developments in Music Therapy Practice: Case study perspectives*. Gilsum, NH: Barcelona Publishers, pp. 134–49.

Carroll, D. (2007a) Portraiture and the role of research: Questions and reflections. *Canadian Journal of Music Therapy*, 32(2), 151–62.

Carroll, D. (2007b) *Children's Use of Personal, Social, and Material Resources to Solve a Music Notational Task: A social constructivist perspective*. (Unpublished doctoral thesis). McGill University, Montreal, Quebec.

Cartwright, D. (2010) *Containing states of mind: Exploring Bion's container model in psychoanalytic psychotherapy*. London: Routledge.

Cassity, M. D. (1976) The influence of a music therapy activity upon peer acceptance, group cohesiveness, and interpersonal relationships of adult psychiatric patients. *Journal of Music Therapy*, 13, 66–76.

Cassity, M. D. (1977) Nontraditional guitar techniques for the educable and trainable mentally retarded residents in music therapy activities. *Journal of Music Therapy*, 14, 39–42.

Cassity, M. D. (1981) The influence of a socially valued skill on peer acceptance in a music therapy group. *Journal of Music Therapy*, 18, 148–54.

Cassity, M. D. and Cassity, J. E. (1994) Psychiatric music therapy assessment and treatment in clinical training facilities. *Journal of Music Therapy*, 31, 2–30.

Cassity, M. D. and Cassity, J. E. (2006) *Multimodal Psychiatric Music Therapy for Adults, Adolescents, and Children: A clinical manual*, 3rd edn. London: Jessica Kingsley Publishers.

Cermak, S., Quintero, E. and Cohen, P. (1980) Developmental age trends in crossing the body midline in normal four through eight-year-old children. *American Journal of Occupational Therapy*, 34, 313–19.

Certification Board for Music Therapists (2011) Music therapy. Retrieved from http://www.cbmt.org/

Cevasco, A. (2010) Effects of the therapist's nonverbal behavior on participation and affect of individuals with Alzheimer's disease during group music therapy sessions. *Journal of Music Therapy*, 47(3), 282–99.

CFA Institute (2005) *Standards of Practice Handbook*, 9th edn. Charlottesville, VA: CFA Institute.

Chadwick, D. and Wacks, K. (2005) *Music Advance Directives: Music choices in later life*. Paper presented at the 11th World Congress, Brisbane, Australia.

Chadwick, D. and Wacks, K. (2011) *Music Assurance: The music living will*. Paper presented at the 13th World Congress, Seoul, South Korea.

Chanda, M. L. and Levitin, D. J. (2013) The neurochemistry of music. *Trends in Cognitive Sciences*, 17(4), 179–93.

Chase, K. (2007) *Land of Stone: Breaking silence through poetry*. Detroit, IL: Wayne State University Press.

Chen, J. L. (2009) The role of auditory and premotor cortex in sensorimotor transformations. *Annals of the New York Academy of Sciences*, 1169, 15–34.

Chhina, C. (2004) Music therapy and psychosocial rehabilitation: Towards a person-centered music therapy model. *Canadian Journal of Music Therapy*, 11(1), 8–30.

Clair, A. A. and Memmott, J. (2008) *Therapeutic Uses of Music with Older Adults*, 2nd edn. Silver Spring, MD: American Music Therapy Association.

Clark, C. and Chadwick, D. (1980) *Clinically Adapted Instruments for the Multiply Handicapped*. St Louis, MO: MMB Music.

Clark, A. (2008) *Supersizing the Mind*. Oxford: Oxford University Press.

Clarke, M. E. (2010) *Climate Change and Human Rights: A case study of the Canadian Inuit and global warming in the Canadian Arctic*. Masters of Laws, University of Toronto, Toronto, ON.

Clarkson, A. (2008) Music therapy with children who have witnessed domestic violence. In S. L. Brooke (ed.) *The Use of the Creative Therapies with Survivors of Domestic Violence*. Springfield, IL: Charles C. Thomas, pp. 136–57.

Claussen, D. and Thaut, M. H. (1997) Music as a mnemonic device for children with learning disabilities. *Canadian Journal of Music Therapy*, 5(1), 55–66.

Clements-Cortés, A. (2004) The use of music in facilitating emotional expression in the terminally ill. *American Journal of Hospice and Palliative Medicine*, 21(4), 255–60.

Cohen, S.; Gilboa, A., Bergstrøm-Nielsen, C., Leder, R. and Milstein, Y. (2012). A multiple perspective approach to graphic notation. Nordic Journal of Music Therapy 21(2).

Cole, S. and Taylor, C. (2008) Free play for all ages. *Children Webmag*, 1 September. Retrieved from http://www.childrenwebmag.com/articles/play-articles/free-play-for-all-ages

Colgin, L. L., Denninger, T., Fyhn, M., Hafting, T., Bonnevie, T., Jensen, O., Moser, M. and Moser, E. I. (2009) Frequency of gamma oscillations routes flow of information in the hippocampus. *Nature,* 462, 353–7.

Collins, K. A. and Dozois, D. J. A. (2008) What are the active ingredients in preventative interventions for depression? *Clinical Psychology: Science and practice*, 15(4), 313–30.

Colwell, C. (2005) The Orff approach to music therapy. *The Orff Echo*, 38(10), 19–21.

Condon, W. S. and Ogston, W. D. (1967) A segmentation of behavior. *Journal of Psychiatric Research*, 221–35.

Cooper, M. L. (2012) A musical analysis of how Mary Priestley implemented the techniques she developed for Analytical Music Therapy. Unpublished Dissertation. Temple University, Philadelphia City, PA.

Corbin, J. and Strauss, A. (2007) *Basics of Qualitative Research: Techniques and procedures for developing grounded theory*. London: Sage Publications.

Cozolino, L. (2006) *The Neuroscience of Human Relationships: Attachment and the human brain*. London: W. W. Norton & Co.

Crade, M. and Llovett, S. (1988) Fetal response to sound stimulation: Preliminary report exploring use of sound stimulation in routine obstetrical ultrasound examinations. *Journal of Ultrasound Medicine*, 7, 499–503.

Craig, J. A. (2012) History of the modes. *Tonal Resources for the Creative Musician*. Anchorage: Cyber School of Music. Retrieved from http://www.jacmuse.com/melodic%20resources/church%20modes/newpage35.htm

Cresswell, J. W. and Clark, V. L. P. (2007) *Designing and Conducting Mixed Methods Research*. London: Sage Publications.

Cresswell, J. W. and Miller, D. (2000) Determining validity in qualitative inquiry. *Theory into Practice*, 39(3), 124–30.

Cripps, T. R., Malik, M., Farrell, T. G. and Camm, A. J. (1991) Prognostic value of reduced heart rate variability after myocardial infarction: Clinical evaluation of a new analysis method. *British Heart Journal*, 65(1), 14–9.

Crits-Christoph, P., Gibbons, M. B. C. and Hearon, B. (2006) Does the alliance cause good outcome? Recommendations for future research on the alliance. *Psychotherapy: Theory, Research, Practice, Training*, 43(3), 280–5.

Crittenden, P. (2007) Care-index: Infants and toddlers. Coding manual. Miami, FL: Family Relations Institute.

Crowe, B. J. (2004) *Music and Soulmaking*. Lanham, MD: Scarecrow Press.

Crowe, B. J. and Rio, R. (2004) Implications of technology in music therapy practice and research for music therapy education: A review of the literature. *Journal of Music Therapy*, 41(4), 282–320.

Csikszentmihalyi, M. (1991) *Flow: The psychology of optimal experience*. New York: Harper and Row.

Curtis, S. L. (1990) Women's issues and music therapists. *Music Therapy Perspectives*, 8, 61–6.

Curtis, S. L. (1996) *Singing subversion, singing soul: Women's voices in feminist music therapy.* (Doctoral dissertation). Concordia University, Montreal, QC. Retrieved from Dissertation Abstracts International, 60 (12–A), 4240.

Damasio, A. R. (2010) *Self Comes to Mind: Constructing the conscious ear*. New York: Pantheon Books.

Darnley-Smith, R. and Patey, H. M. (2003) *Music Therapy*. London: Sage.

Das, K. (2011) *The Way of Music: Creating sounds connections in music therapy*. Denton, TX: Sarsen.

Das, K. and Matney, B. (2011) A taxonomy of drumming experiences [Web log message]. Retrieved from http://musictherapydrumming.com/a-taxonomy-of-drumming-experiences-2/

Davies, D. (1996) Towards a model of gay affirmative therapy. In D. Davies and C. Neal (eds) *Pink Therapy: A guide for counsellors and therapists working with lesbian, gay and bisexual clients*. Buckingham: Open University Press.

Davis, W. B. (2003) Ira Maximillian Altshuler: Psychiatrist and pioneer music therapist. *Journal of Music Therapy*, 40(2), 151–68.

Davis, W. B., Gfeller, K. F. and Thaut, M. H. (eds) (1999) *An Introduction to Music Therapy Theory and Practice*, 2nd edn. Boston, MA: McGraw-Hill College.

Davis, W. B., Gfeller, K. F. and Thaut, M. H. (2008) *An Introduction to Music Therapy Theory and Practice*, 3rd edn. Silver Spring, MD: AMTA.

De Backer, J. (1993) Containment in music therapy. In T. Wigram and M. Heal (eds) *Music Therapy in Health and Education*. London: Jessica Kingsley.

De Backer, J. (2005) *The Transition from Sensorial Play to Musical Form by Psychotic Patients in a Music Therapeutic Process*. (Unpublished doctoral dissertation). Aalborg University, Aalborg, Denmark.

De Backer, J. (2008) A research report detailing the transition form sensorial play to musical form by psychotic patients. *Nordic Journal of Music Therapy*, 17(2), 89–104.

De Backer, J. (2011) Het therapeutisch bewogen worden in een muzikale ruimte. In M. De Hert, D. De Wachter, G. Pieters, L. Van Bouwel and R. Vermote (eds) *Fervet Opus: Actuele trends in de geestelijke gezondheidszorg*. Berchem: Epo, pp. 88–95.

Decker-Voigt, H. and Weymann, E. (2009) *Lexikon Musiktherapie*. Bern: Verlag Hogrefe.

del Campo, P. (2002) *El psiquismo creador y Musicoterapia*. Barcelona: Universidad de Valladolid.

Delrieu, A. (1997) *Sigmund Freud: Index thématique*. Paris: Économica.

DeNora, T. (2000) *Music in Everyday Life*. Cambridge: Cambridge University Press.

DeRubeis, R. J., Brotman, M. A. and Gibbons, C. J. (2005) A conceptual and methodological analysis of the nonspecifics argument. *Clinical Psychology: Science and Practice*, 12, 174–83.

Dietrich, A. (2003) Functional neuroanatomy of altered states of consciousness: The transient hypofrontality hypothesis. *Consciousness and Cognition*, 12(2), 231–56.

Dietrich, A. (2010) A review of EEG, ERP, and neuroimaging studies of creativity and insight. *Psychological Bulletin*, 136(5), 822–48.

Dileo, C. (2000) *Ethical Thinking in Music Therapy*. Cherry Hill, NJ: Jeffrey Books.

Dileo, C. (2011) Final notes: Therapeutic uses of the voice with imminently dying patients. In F. A. Baker and S. Uhlig (eds) *Voicework in Music Therapy*. London: Jessica Kingsley Publishers, pp. 321–32.

Dileo, C. and Dneaster, D. (2005) Introduction: State of the art. In C. Dileo and J. V. Loewy (eds) *Music Therapy at the End-of-life*. Cherry Hill, NJ: Jeffrey Books, pp. xix–xxvii.

Dileo, C. and Loewy, J. (eds) (2005) *Music Therapy at the End-of-life*. Cherry Hill, NJ: Jeffrey Books.

Dileo Maranto, C. (ed.) (1993) *Music Therapy: International perspectives*. Pipersville, PA: Jeffrey Books.

Dillard, L. M. (2006) Musical countertransference experiences of music therapists: A phenomenological study. *The Arts in Psychotherapy*, 31, 208–17. doi: 10.1016/j.aip.2006.01.002

Dimoff, T. (2008) Improvisation games: Creating spontaneous music in groups. Retrieved from http://plato.acadiau.ca/courses/educ/Reid/Games/Game_descriptions/Improvisation_Games.html

Dixon, M. (2002) Music and human rights. In J. P. Sutton (ed.) *Music, Music Therapy, and Trauma*. London: Jessica Kingsley, pp. 119–32.

Dixon-Woods, M. and Fitzpatrick, R. (2001) Qualitative research in systematic reviews has established a place for itself. *British Medical Journal*, 323, 765–6.

Donaghy, M. (2009) *Brain's Diseases of the Nervous System*, 12th edn. Oxford: Oxford University Press.

Dowling, W. J. and Harwood, D. L. (1986) *Music Cognition*. New York: Academic Press.

Duncan, B. L., Miller, S. D. and Sparks, J. A. (2000) *The Heroic Client: A revolutionary way to improve effectiveness through client-directed, outcome-informed therapy*. San Francisco, CA: Jossey-Bass.

Dunn, B., Hearns, M., Jackert, L., Rio, R. and Winnwalker, J. (2010) You are a song. *Daughters of Harriet* [CD]. Hollywood, CA: Studio Recording.

Edwards, J. (2011) *Music Therapy and Parent–Infant Bonding*. New York: Oxford University Press.

Edwards, J. (2012) We need to talk about epistemology: Orientations, meaning, and interpretation within music therapy research. *Journal of Music Therapy*, 49, 372–94.

Elligan, D. (2004) *Rap Therapy: A practical guide for communicating with young adults through rap music*. New York: Kensington.

Elliott, D. J. (1995) *Music Matters: A new philosophy of music education*. New York: Oxford University Press.

Engen, R. L. (2005) The singer's breath: Implications for treatment of persons with emphysema. *Journal of Music Therapy*, 42(1), 20–48.

Erkkilä, J., Gold, C., Fachner, J., Ala-Ruona, E., Punkanen, M. and Vanhala, M. (2008) The effect of improvisational music therapy on the treatment of depression: Protocol for a randomised controlled trial. *BMC Psychiatry*, 8(50), 1–9. doi: 10.1186/1471-244X-8-50.

Erkskine, R. G. (1998) Attunement and involvement: Therapeutic responses to relational needs. *International Journal of Psychotherapy*, 3, 325–344.

Ernst, E. and Randl, J. I. (1998) Complementary therapies for depression. *Archives of General Psychiatry*, 55, 1026–32.

Eschen, J. T. (ed.) (2002) *Analytical Music Therapy*. London: Jessica Kingsley.

Farnsworth, P. R. (1958) *The Social Psychology of Music*. New York: The Dryden Press.

Fausto-Sterling, A. (2000) *Sexing the Body: Gender politics and construction of sexuality*. New York: Basic Books.

Federico, G. F. (2005) *Focal Music Therapy in Obstetric Area, Pregnancy*. Paper presented at the XI World Congress of Music Therapy, Brisbane, Australia. http://gabrielfederico.com/articles/australia2005.pdf

Federico, G. F. (2011) *Procedure CIMI: Conducted improvisation with musical instruments with pregnant women, in focal music therapy in obstetrics (FMTO)*. Paper presented at the Third International Music Therapy Research Conference, Waterloo, ON. http://gabrielfederico.com/articles/canada2011.pdf

Federico, G. F. and Whitwell, G. E. (2001) Music therapy and pregnancy. *Journal of Prenatal and Perinatal Psychology and Health*, 15(2), 299–311.

Feil, N. (2002) *The Validation Breakthrough: Simple techniques for communicating with people with 'Alzheimer's-type dementia'*, 2nd edn. Baltimore, MD: Health Professions Press.

Feil, N. and de Klerk-Rubin, V. (1982/1992) *V/F Validation: The Feil method*, rev. edn. Shaker Heights, OH: Edward Feil Productions.

Ferraiolo, S. (2004) You have been framed: Maternity and the male psychotherapist. In M. Luca (ed.) *The Therapeutic Frame in the Clinical Context: Integrative perspective*. East Sussex: Brunner-Routledge, pp. 67–85.

Fick, S. and Shilts, E. (2006) This is your brain on music: Mapping mental activity reveals that music stimulates the brain in the same way food, sex, and drugs do. *Canadian Geographic*, Jan/Feb.

Finlay, L. and Gough, B. (2003) *Reflexivity: A practical guide for researchers in health and social sciences*. Oxford: Blackwell Publishing.

Fiorini, H. (2002) *Teoría y Técnica de Psicoterapias*. Buenos Aires: Nueva Visión.

Fiorini, H. (ed.) (2010) *Creative Psyche*. AgruArte: Vitoria-Gasteiz.

Fitzgerald, M. (1998) Child psychoanalytic psychotherapy. *Advances in Psychiatric Treatment*, 4, 18–24.

Fitzgerald, M. J. (2012) *Clinical Neuroanatomy and Neuroscience*, 6th edn. New York: Elsevier.

Fogerty, D. and Humes, L. E. (2012) The role of vowel and consonant fundamental frequency, envelope, and temporal fine structure cues to the intelligibility of words and sentences. Bloomington, *Journal of the Acoustical Society of America*, 131(2), 1490–501. doi: 10.1121/1.3676696

Fogerty, D. and Kewley-Port, D. (2008) Investigating the consonant-vowel boundary: Perceptual contributions to sentence intelligibility. *Proceedings of Meetings on Acoustics, Vol. 2, Speech Communication*. New Orleans, LA: Acoustical Society of America. doi: http://dx.doi.org/10.1121/1.2972133

Forinash, M. (ed.) (2001) *Music Therapy Supervision*. Gilsum, NH: Barcelona Publishers.

Fornazzari, L., Castle, T., Nadkarni, S., Ambrose, M., Apanasiewicz, N. and Phillips, F. (2006) Preservation of episodic musical memory in a pianist with Alzheimer disease. *Neurology*, 66(4), 610–11.

Foulkes, S. H. (1968/1990) Group dynamic processes and group analysis (1968). In S. H. Foulkes (ed.) *Selected Papers of S. H. Foulkes: Psychoanalysis and group process* (E. Foulkes, ed.). London: Karnac Books, pp. 47–75.

Foulkes, S. H. (1973/1990) The group as matrix of the individual's mental life. In L. R. Wolberg and E. K. Schwartz (eds) *Group Therapy: An overview*. New York: Intercontinental Medical Book Corporation, 1973, pp. 211–20. (Reprinted in S.H. Foulkes, Selected Papers, Psychoanalysis and Group-analysis, edited by Foulkes, E.T. London: Karnac Books, 1990).

Fox, J. (1997) *Poetic Medicine: The healing art of poem making*. New York: Jeremy Tarcher.

Frank, R. M. (2007) Introduction: Sociocultural situatedness. In T. Ziemke, J. Zlatev and R. M. Frank (eds) *Body, Language, and Mind,* Vol. 2: Embodiment, pp. 1–18. Berlin: de Gruyter.

Frankl, V. (2004) *Man's Search for Meaning: An introduction to logotherapy*. Boston, MA: Beacon.

Freud, S. (1914/1957) *On the History of the Psycho-Analytic Movement*, standard edn., vol. 7. London: Hogarth Press & Institute of Psycho-Analysis.

Freud, S. (1975) *Civilization and its Discontents*, translated by J. Riviere, rev. edn., vol. 17. London: Hogarth Press & Institute of Psycho-Analysis.

Fujioka, T., Trainor, L. J., Large, E. W. and Ross, B. (2009) Beta and gamma rhythms in human auditory cortex during musical beat processing. *Annals of the New York Academy of Sciences*, 1169, 89–92.

Fuhrman, R. (2002) Poetry therapy as a tool for strength-based practice. *Advances in Social Work*, 3, 147–57.

Fuster, J. (2008) *The Prefrontal Cortex*, 4th edn. New York: Academic Press.

Gaidos, S. (2010) More than a feeling: Emotionally evocative, yes, but music goes much deeper. *Science News*, 178(4), 24–9.

Gallagher, L. M., Lagman, R., Walsh, D., Davis, M. B. and LeGrand, S. B. (2006) The clinical effects of music therapy in palliative medicine. *Supportive Care Cancer*, 14, 859–66.

Gallese, V. (2006) Intentional attunement: A neurophysiological perspective on social cognition and its disruption in autism. *Cognitive Brain Research*, 1079, 15–24.

Gardner, S. E. B. (2008) Iyómex, Éyqwlha, Yú: Wqwlha, Language as musical space, an aesthetic approach to research. *Voices: A world forum for music therapy*, 8(3). Retrieved from https://normt.uib.no/index.php/voices/article/view/412/336

Gardstrom, S. C. (2008) Music therapy as noninvasive treatment: Who says? *Nordic Journal of Music Therapy*, 17(2), 142–54.

Garnets, L. D. and Kimmel, D. C. (2003) Lesbian, gay male and bisexual dimensions in the psychology study of human diversity. In L. D. Garnets and D. C. Kimmel (eds) *Psychological Perspectives on Lesbian, Gay, and Bisexual Experiences*, 2nd edn. New York: Columbia University Press Books.

Garoian, C. (1999) *Performing Pedagogy: Toward an art of politics*. Albany, NY: State University of New York Press.

Garred, R. (2006) *Music as Therapy: A dialogical perspective*. Gilsum, NH: Barcelona Publishers.

Gaston, E. T. (ed.) (1968) *Music in Therapy*. New York: Macmillan.

Gentner, D. and Colhoun, J. (2010) Analogical processes in human thinking and learning. In B. Glatzeder, V. Goel and A. von Müller (eds) *On Thinking. Volume 2: Towards a Theory of Thinking: Building blocks for a conceptual framework*. Berlin: Springer, pp. 35–48.

Gerdner, L. A. (2000) Effects of individualized versus classical 'relaxation' music on the frequency of agitation in elderly persons with Alzheimer's disease and related disorders. *International Psychogeriatrics*, 12(1), 49–65.

Gfeller, K. E. (1983) Musical mnemonics as an aid to retention with normal and learning disabled students. *Journal of Music Therapy*, 20(4), 179–89.

Gfeller, K. E. (2008) Music: A human phenomenon and therapeutic tool. In W. B. Davis, K. E. Gfeller and M. H. Thaut (eds) *An Introduction to Music Therapy: Theory and practice*, 3rd edn. Silver Spring, MD: American Music Therapy Association, pp. 41–76.

Gfeller, K. E., Christ, A., Knutson, J., Witt, S. and Mehr, M. (2003) The effect of familiarity and complexity on appraisal of complex songs by cochlear implant recipients and normal hearing adults. *Journal of Music Therapy*, 40(2), 78–112.

Gibson, J. J. (1986) *The Ecological Approach to Visual Perception*. Hillsdale, NJ: Lawrence Erlbaum Associates.

Giddens, A. (1984) *The Constitution of Society: Outline of the theory of structuration*. Cambridge: Cambridge University Press.

Gilbertson, S. (2009) A reference standard bibliography: Music therapy with children who have experienced traumatic brain injury. *Music and Medicine*, 1(2), 129–39.

Gilbertson, S. and Aldridge, D. (2008) *Music Therapy and Traumatic Brain Injury: A light on a dark night*. London: Jessica Kingsley.

Glaser, B. G. and Strauss, A. L. (2009) *The Discovery of Grounded Theory: Strategies for qualitative research*, 4th edn. Piscataway, NJ: Aldine Transaction.

Go, T. (2007) Medical music therapy based on baby science (baby science-based music therapy) and assistive technology for children. *Current Pediatric Reviews*, 3(3), 198.

Goff, T. (2012) The soundtrack of life. *TREK Online*, January/February. Retrieved from http://trekmagazine.alumni.ubc.ca/2012/januaryfebruary-2012/features/the-soundtrack-of-life/

Gold, C., Rolvsjord, R., Aarø, L. E., Aarre, T., Tjemsland, L. and Stige, B. (2005) Resource-oriented music therapy for psychiatric patients with low therapy motivation: Protocol for a randomised controlled trial. *BMC Psychiatry*, 5(39), 1–8. doi: 10.1186/1471-244X-5-39

Gold, C., Heldal, T. O., Dable, T. and Wigram, T. (2005) Music therapy for schizophrenia or schizophrenia-like illnesses. *Cochrane Database of Systematic Reviews* (2). doi: 10.1002/14651858.CD004025.pub2

Gold, C., Wigram, T. and Elefant, C. (2006) Music therapy for autistic spectrum disorder. *Cochrane Database of Systematic Reviews* (2). doi: 10.1002/ 14651858.CD004381.pub2

Goldfried, M. R. and Davila, J. (2005) The role of relationship and technique in therapeutic change. *Psychotherapy: Theory, Research, Practice, Training*, 42(4), 421–30.

Goodale, M. (2009) *Surrendering to Utopia: An anthropology of human rights*. Stanford, CA: Stanford University Press.

Goodheart, H. K. (2001) Temple University to honor three faculty members for their outstanding achievement. Temple University Office of News and Media Relations. Retrieved from https://www.temple.edu/news_media/hkg395.html

Goodman, K. D. (1989) Music therapy assessment of emotionally disturbed children. *The Arts in Psychotherapy*, 16, 179–92.

Goodman, K. D. (2007) *Music Therapy Groupwork with Special Needs Children: The evolving process*. Springfield, IL: Charles C. Thomas.

Gordon, E. E. (2005) *Preparatory Audiation, Audition, and Music Learning Theory: A handbook of a comprehensive music learning sequence*. Chicago, IL: GIA Publications.

Goren-Bar, A. (1997) The 'creation axis' in expressive therapies. *The Arts in Psychotherapy*, 24(5), 411–18.

Greenspan, S. and Weider, S. (1998) *The Child with Special Needs: Encouraging intellectual and emotional growth*. Reading, MA: Perseus.

Greenwald, D. F., Harder, D. W., Ritzler, B. A., Strauss, J. S. and Kokes, R. F. (1988) The Last–Weiss Rorschach Ego-Strength Scale as a prognostic measure for psychiatric outpatients. *Perceptual Motor Skills*, 67(1), 199–207.

Grob, H. M. (1981) Music therapy utilizing paraverbal techniques. In R. F. DiCuio and R. B. Kugel (eds) *Into the Light: Helping people with handicaps at Flower Hospital*. New York: New York Medical Publishing and Flower Hospital, pp. 95–6.

Grob, H. M. (1998) Paraverbal psychomotor techniques in neurologic habilitation and rehabilitation. In C. M. Tomaino (ed.) *Clinical Applications of Music in Neurologic Rehabilitation*. St Louis, MO: MMB, pp. 37–40.

Grocke, D. E. and Wigram, T. (2007a) *Receptive Methods in Music Therapy*. London: Jessica Kingsley Publishers.

Grocke, D. E. and Wigram, T. (2007b) Selecting music for receptive methods in music therapy. In D. E. Grocke and T. Wigram (eds) *Receptive Methods in Music Therapy: Techniques and clinical applications for music therapy clinicians, educators, and students*. London: Jessica Kingsley, pp. 45–60.

Grocke, D. E. and Ip-Winfield, V. (2011) Group music therapy methods in cross-cultural aged care practice in Australia. *Australian Journal of Music Therapy*, 22, 59–78.

Guétin, S., Giniès, P., Blayac, J. P. and Eledjam, J.-J. (2005) Une nouvelle technique contrôlée de musicothérapie dans la prise en charge des douleurs viscérales aiguës et chroniques. *Douleurs et Analgésie*, 1, 19–25.

Guétin, S., Charras, K., Berard, A., Arbus, C., Perthelon, P., Blanc, F., and Leger, J. M. (2012) An overview of the use of music therapy in the context of Alzheimer's disease: A report of a French expert group *Dementia*, April 8, 1–16. doi: 10.1177/ 1471301212438290

Gutheil, T. G. and Brodsky, A. (2008) *Preventing Boundary Violations in Clinical Practice*. New York: Guilford Press.

Hadley, S. (ed.) (1998) *Psychodynamic Music Therapy: Case studies*. Gilsum, NH: Barcelona Publishers.

Hadley, S. (2001) Exploring relationships between Mary Priestley's life and work. *Nordic Journal of Music Therapy*, 10(2), 116–31.

Hadley, S. (2005) Psychiatric music therapy in the community: The legacy of Florence Tyson [Supplemental material]. *Nordic Journal of Music Therapy*, 5 March. [Review of the book *Psychiatric Music Therapy in the Community: The legacy of Florence Tyson* edited by M. G. McGuire] Retrieved from http://njmt.b.uib.no/2005/03/04/psychiatric-music-therapy-in-the-community-the-legacy-of-florence-tyson/

Hadley, S. (ed.) (2006) *Feminist Perspectives in Music Therapy*. Gilsum, NH: Barcelona Publishers.

Hadley, S. and Yancy, G. (eds) (2011) *Therapeutic Uses of Rap and Hip-hop*. New York: Routledge.

Hakomäki, H. (2009) Storycomposing: An interactive and creative way to express one's own musical inventions. In W. C. Turgeon (ed.) *Creativity and the Child: Interdisciplinary perspectives*. Oxford: Inter-Disciplinary Press.

Hall, E. T. (1992) Improvisation as an acquired, multilevel process. *Ethnomusicology*, 36(2), 223–35.

Hallam, S. and MacDonald, R. (2008) The effects of music in community and educational settings. In S. Hallam, I. Cross and M. Thaut (eds) *The Oxford Handbook of Music Psychology*. Oxford: Oxford University Press, pp. 471–80.

Hamel, P. M. (1978) *Through Music to the Self: How to appreciate and experience music anew*, translated by P. Lemesurier. Shaftesbury, England: Element Books.

Hammersley, M. and Atkinson, P. (1983) *Ethnography, Principles in Practice*. London: Routledge.

Haneishi, E. (2005) Juliette Alvin: Her legacy for music therapy in Japan. *Journal of Music Therapy*, 42(4), 273–95.

Hanser, S. B. (1999) *The New Music Therapist's Handbook*. Boston, MA: Berklee Press.

Hanser, S. B., Butterfield-Whitcomb, J., Kawata, M. and Collins, B. (2011) Home-based music strategies with individuals who have dementia and their family caregivers. *Journal of Music Therapy*, 48(1), 2–27.

Hanson-Abromeit, D., Fisher, C. and Merz, E. (2011) *Preventive Music Therapy for Children Living in Poverty*. Pre-conference 5-hour continuing music therapy education course, American Music Therapy Association 12th Annual Conference, Atlanta, GA.

Hanson, W. E., Creswell, J. W., Clark, V. L. P., Petska, K. S. and Creswell, J. D. (2005) Mixed methods research designs in counseling psychology. *Journal of Counseling Psychology*, 52(2), 224–35.

Harré, R. and Secord, P. (1971) *The Explanation of Social Behaviour*. London: Blackwell.

Harrington, L. (2000) Introduction. In R. F. Harrington (ed.) *The Soul Solution*. Galena Bay, BC: White Oak Press, pp. i–v.

Harrison, S., Cooke, M., Moyle, W., Shum, D. and Murfield, J. E. (2010) Development of a music intervention protocol and its effect on participant engagement: Experiences from a randomised controlled trial with older people with dementia. *Arts and Health*, 2(2), 125–39.

Hawkins, P. and Shohet, R. (2000) *Supervision in the Helping Professions*, 2nd edn. Buckingham: Open University Press.

Heal, M. and Wigram, T. (eds) (1993) *Music Therapy in Health and Education*. London: Jessica Kingsley.

Heimann, P. (1950) On counter-transference. *International Journal of Psychoanalysis*, 31, 81–4.

Heimlich, E. P. (1972) Paraverbal techniques in the therapy of childhood communication disorders. *International Journal of Child Psychotherapy*, 1(1), 65–83.

Heimlich, E. P. and Mark, A. J. (1990) *Paraverbal Communication with Children* New York: Plenum Press.

Heirman, L. (1971) Eurythmy as an art. In E. Pouderoyen (ed.) *Eurythmy*. Nortridge, CA: Eurythmy Association of Southern California.

Hendon, C. and Bohon, L. M. (2007) Hospitalized children's mood differences during play and music therapy. *Child: Care, Health and Development*, 34, 141–4.

Hepper, P. G. and Shahidullah, B. S. (1994) Development of fetal hearing. *Archives of Disease in Childhood*, 71, F81–7.

Herman, F. and Smith, J. C. (1988) *Accentuate the Positive: Expressive arts for children with disabilities*. Toronto, ON: Jimani Publications.

Herman, F. and Smith, J. C. (1992) *Creatability: Creative arts for preschool children with special needs*. Tucson, AZ: Jimani Publications.

Heslop, A. (1992) Qualities of the effective counsellor. *The Child Care Worker*, 10(6), 10–11.

Hillecke, T., Nickel, A. and Bolay, H. V. (2005) Scientific perspectives on music therapy. *Annals of the New York Academy of Sciences*, 1060, 271–82.

Hillecke, T. and Wilker, F. W. (2007) Ein heuristisches Wirkfaktorenmodell der Musiktherapie. *Verhaltenstherapie and Verhaltensmedizin*, 28(1), 62–85.

Hoffman, L. (2004) Existential therapy. Retrieved from http://www.existential-therapy.com

Hoffman, S. and Laub, B. (2006) *Innovative Interventions in Psychotherapy*. Boca Raton, FL: Universal Publishers.

Horne-Thompson, A. (2003) Expanding from hospital to home based care: Implications for music therapists working in palliative care. *Australian Journal of Music Therapy*, 14, 38–49.

Hugo, V. (2007) *Hugo's Works: William Shakespeare*, Vol. 19. Rockville, MD: Wildside Press.

Hull, A. (2012) Drum circles defined. Remo, Inc. Retrieved from http://www.remo.com/portal/pages/drum_circles/defined/Drum+Circles+Defined+What+is+a+Drum+Cicle.html

Hunt, W. and Issacharoff, A. (1977) Heinrich Racker and counter-transference theory. *Journal of the American Academy of Psychoanalysis and Dynamic Psychiatry*, 5, 95–105.

Husserl, E. (1969) *The Phenomenology of Internal Time-Consciousness (1893–1917)*, translated by R. Boehm. The Hague: Martinus Nijhoff.

Huxley, J. and Haddon, A. C. (1936) *We Europeans: A survey of 'racial' problems*. New York and London: Harper.

Intveen, A. (2007) Musical instruments in anthroposophical music therapy with reference to Rudolf Steiner's model of the threefold human being. *Voices: A world forum for music therapy*, 7(3). Retrieved from https://normt.uib.no/index.php/voices/article/viewArticle/547/408

Intveen, A. (2010) 'The piano is a wooden box with false teeth': Perspectives in anthroposophical music therapy as revealed through interviews with two expert practitioners *The Arts in Psychotherapy*, 37, 370–7.

Iwanaga, M. and Kobayashi, A. (2005) Heart rate variability with repetitive exposure to music. *Biological Psychology*, 70(1), 61–6.

Izquierdo, M. A., Oliver, D. L. and Malmierca, M. S. (2009) Mecanismos de plasticidad (funcional y dependiente de actividad) en el cerebro auditivo adulto y en desarrollo. *Revista de Neurología*, 48, 421–9.

Jackert, L. and Rio, R. (2007) *Introducing Strength-based Improvisation*. Paper presented at the Western Region AMTA Conference Training Manual.

Jacobsen, S. and Wigram, T. (2007) Music therapy for the assessment of parental competencies for children in need of care. *Nordic Journal of Music Therapy*, 16, 129–43.

Jadad, A. R. and Enkin, M. W. (2007) *Randomized Controlled Trials: Questions, answers, and musings*, 2nd edn. Malden, MA: Blackwell Publishing.

James, S. (1999) *Roots and Blues Fingerstyle Guitar*. San Anselmo, CA: String Letter Publishing.

Janata, P. (2005) Brain networks that track musical structure. *Annals of the New York Academy of Sciences*, 1060, 111–24.

Janata, P. and Grafton, S. T. (2003) Swinging in the brain: Shared neural substrates for behaviors related to sequencing and music. *Nature Neuroscience*, 6, 682–7.

Jauset, J. Á. (2010) *Sonida, Música y Espiritualidad: Un camina científico hacia la unidad*. Madrid: Ediciones Gaia.

Jauset, J. Á. (2011) *Apia de sonido ¿Ciencia o dogma?* Barcelona: Luciérnaga.

Jahn-Langenberg, M. (2003) Harmony and Dissonance in Conflict: Psychoanalytically Informed Music Therapy with a Psychosomatic Patient, in S. Hadley (ed.) *Psychodynamic Music Therapy: Case Studies*, Gilsum, NH: Barcelona Publishers.

Lazarus, P. A. and Roslyn, F. M. (2003) The arts in medicine: Setting up and evaluating a new special study module at Leicester Warwick Medical School. *Medical Education*, 37, 553–59.

Jensen, B. (1999) Music therapy with psychiatric in-patients. In T. Wigram and J. De Backer (eds) *Clinical Applications of Music Therapy in Psychiatry*. London: Jessica Kingsley, pp. 34–60.

Jeppe, Z. (2006) Dance/movement and music in improvisational concert: A model for psychotherapy. *The Arts in Psychotherapy*, 33, 371–82.

Johnson, R. E. (1981) E. Thayer Gaston: Leader in scientific thought on music in therapy and education. *Journal of Research in Music Education*, 29(4), 279–86. doi: 10.2307/3345004

Johnson, M. (2007) *The Meaning of the Body: Aesthetics of human understanding*. Chicago, IL: The University of Chicago Press.

Johnsson, K. O. (2001) The roles and functions of cutaneous mechanoreceptors. *Current Opinion in Neurobiology*, 11, 455–61.

Jordenson, D. L. (1989) *Methods of Collecting Information. Participant Observation: A methodology for human studies*, 15. Thousand Oaks, CA: SAGE Publications.

Jourt Pineau, C. (2012) La musicothérapie en oncologie. *Revue de Musicothérapie, April.*

Juslin, P. N., Liljeström, S., Västfjäll, D. and Lundqvist, L.-O. (2010) How does music evoke emotions? Exploring the underlying mechanisms. In P. N. Juslin and J. Sloboda (eds) *Handbook of Music and Emotion: Theory, research, applications*. New York: Oxford University Press, pp. 605–42.

Kannengiesser, S. (2009) *Sprachentwicklungstörungen: Grundlagen, Diagnostik und Therapie*. Munich: Urban & Fischer Verlag.

Karkkainen, M. and Mitsui, J. (2006) The effects of sound based vibration treatment on the human mind and body: the physioacoustic method. *Journal of International Society of Life Information Science*, 24(1), 155–59.

Karkou, V. and Sanderson, P. (2006) *Arts Therapies: A research-based map of the field.* Edinburgh: Elsevier.

Kay, L. D. (1981) Music therapy activities for the severely and profoundly multiply handicapped child or adult. *Voices of the Lakes [Newsletter of the Great Lakes Regional Chapter, NAMT]*, 25, 26–30.

Kenny, C. (1985) Music: A whole systems approach. *Music Therapy*, 5(1), 3–11.

Kenny, C. (1989) *The Field of Play: A guide for the theory and practice of music therapy.* Atascadero, CA: Ridgeview Publishing.

Kenny, C. (2006) *Music and Life in the Field of Play: An anthology.* Gilsum, NH: Barcelona Publishers.

Kenny, C. B. (1982) *The Mythic Artery.* Atascadero, CA: Ridgeview Publishing.

Kenny, C. B. (1999) Beyond this point there be dragons: Developing a general theory in music therapy. *Nordic Journal of Music Therapy*, 8(2), 127–36.

Keyes, E. (1973) *Toning: The creative power of the voice.* Marina del Ray, CA: DeVorss & Co.

Kirkland, K. (2004) *A Grim Fairy Tale: A mythopoetic discourse on taboo, trauma, and anti-oppressive pedagogy.* (Unpublished doctoral dissertation). University of British Columbia, Vancouver, BC.

Kirkland, K., Fortuna, M. C., Kelson, E. and Phinney, A. (2013) Music, spirituality, and meaning: A mixed methods study of a combined music therapy and spiritual care group for persons with dementia. *Canadian Journal of Music Therapy*, 19(1).

Kitchen, K. (2005) Beyond therapeutic models: Do therapists know what clients really want? *CrossCurrents*, 9(1), 1–17.

Kitwood, T. (1997a) *Dementia Reconsidered: The person comes first.* Buckingham: Open University Press.

Kitwood, T. (1997b) The experience of dementia. *Aging and Mental Health*, 1(1), 13–22.

Klein, M. (1961/1984) Narrative of a child analysis. In R. Money-Kyrle (ed.) *The Writings of Melanie Klein*, 4(55). New York: Free Press.

Kline, J. A. (1996) Listening effectively. Retrieved from http://www.au.af.mil/au/awc/awcgate/kline-listen/b10toc.htm

Kline, J. A. (2002) *Listening Effectively: Achieving high standards in communications.* Upper Saddle River, NJ: Prentice Hall.

Kohl, H. (1992) *From Archetype to Zeitgeist: Powerful ideas for powerful thinking.* Boston: Little, Brown & Company.

Kohut, H. and Levarie, S. (1950/1978) On the enjoyment of listening to music. In P. H. Omstein (ed.) *The Search for the Self: Selected writings of Heinz Kohut, 1978–1981.* Madison, CT: International Universities Press, pp. 135–8.

Körlin, D. (2007–2008) Music breathing: Breath grounding and modulation of the Bonny Method of Guided Imagery and Music (BMGIM): Theory, method and consecutive cases. *Journal of the Association for Music and Imagery*, 11, 79–113.

Körlin, D. (2010) *Music Listening, Imagery and Creativity in Psychiatry: Guided Imagery and Music (GIM) and Creative Arts Therapies (CATs) in stress disorders.* Saarbrücken: Lambert Academic Publishing.

Kovach, A. M. S. (1985) Shamanism and Guided Imagery and Music: A comparison. *Journal of Music Therapy*, 22, 154–65.

Kraemer, S. (2006) Something happens: Elements of therapeutic change. *Clinical Child Psychology and Psychiatry*, 11(2), 239–48.

Krakouer, L., Houghton, S., Douglas, G. and West, J. (2001) The efficacy of music therapy in effecting change in persons with cerebral palsy. *International Journal of Psychosocial Rehabilitation*, 6, 29–37.

Krauss, T. and Galloway, H. (1982) Melodic intonation therapy with language delayed apraxic children. *Journal of Music Therapy*, 9, 102–13.

Kreutz, G. and Lotze, M. (2007) Neuroscience of music and emotion. In W. Gruhn and F. Rauscher (eds) *Neurosciences in Music Pedagogy*. Hauppauge, NY: Nova Science Publishers, pp. 143–67.

Kris, E. (1952) *Psychoanalytic Explorations in Art*. Oxford: International Universities Press.

Krout, R. E. (2008) Assessing and using emerging adaptive electronic music technology to facilitate creative client expression in music therapy. *New Zealand Journal of Music Therapy*, 6, 27–46.

Krumhansl, C. L. (2000) Rhythm and pitch in music cognition. *Psychological Bulletin*, 126, 159–79.

Lakoff, G. and Johnson, M. L. (1980) *Metaphors We Live By*. Chicago, IL: University of Chicago Press.

Lamont, A. (2009) Music in the school years. In S. Hallam, I. Cross and M. Thaut (eds) *Oxford Handbook of Music Psychology*. Oxford: Oxford University Press.

Langer, S. K. (1942) *Philosophy in a New Key: A study in the symbolism of reason, rite and art*. New York: New American Library of World Literature.

Larson, T. (2002) *History and Tradition of Jazz*. Dubuque, IA: Kendall/Hunt Publishing.

Lashley, K. S. (1951) The problems of serial order in behavior. In L. A. Jeffress (ed.) *Cerebral Mechanisms in Behavior*. New York: Wiley, pp. 112–36.

Lawrence-Lightfoot, S. and Hoffman-Davis, J. (1997) *The Art and Science of Portraiture*. San Francisco, CA: Jossey-Bass.

Lazarus, A. (1981) *The Practice of Multimodal Therapy*. New York: McGraw-Hill.

Lecanuet, J.-P. (1996) The fetal stage. In I. Deliège and J. Sloboda (eds) *Musical Beginnings: Origins and development of musical competence*. New York: Oxford University Press, pp. 3–36.

Lee, C. (2003) *The Architecture of Aesthetic Music Therapy*. Gilsum, NH: Barcelona Publishers.

Lee, C. and Houde, M. (2011) *Improvising in Styles: A workbook for music therapists, educators and musicians*. Gilsum, NH: Barcelona Publishers.

Lefebvre, C. (1991) All her 'yesterdays:' An adolescent's search for a better today through music. In K. E. Bruscia (ed.) *Case Studies in Music Therapy*. Gilsum, NH: Barcelona Publishers, pp. 220–30.

Lehikoinen, P. (1996) *Physioacoustic Sound in Stimulation of Cell Membranes*. Helsinki: Next Wave.

Lehikoinen, P. (1997) The physioacoustic method. In T. Wigram and C. Dileo (eds) *Music, Vibration, and Health*. Cherry Hill, NJ: Jeffrey Books, pp. 209–15.

Leisenring, J. (2001) 'Rupe' (Wayne Ruppenthal). *Jazz Ambassadors Magazine*. Retrieved from http://www.kcjazzambassadors.com/issues/1997–02/salute.html

Leite, T. (2003) Music psychotherapy in groups with acute psychotic patients. *International Journal of Psychotherapy*, 8(2), 117–28.

Lerdahl, F. and Jackendoff, R. (1983) *A Generative Theory of Tonal Music*. Cambridge, MA: MIT Press.

Lerner, P. M. (1998) *Psychoanalytic Perspectives on the Rorschach*. Hillsdale, NJ: The Analytic Press.

Leung, M. (2008) Collaboration between music therapy and speech pathology in a pediatric rehabilitation setting. *Voices: A world forum for music therapy*, 8(3). Retrieved from https://normt.uib.no/index.php/voices/article/view/417/341

Lev, A. I. (2005) Psychotherapy. In C. J. Summers, (ed.) *glbtq: An encyclopedia of gay, lesbian, bisexual, transgender and queer culture*. Chicago, IL: glbtq, Inc. Retrieved from http://www.glbtq.com/social–sciences/psychotherapy.html

Levitin, D. J. (2006) *This is Your Brain on Music: The science of a human obsession*. New York: Dutton.

Levitin, D. J. (2009) The neural correlates of temporal structure in music. *Music and Medicine*, 1(1), 9–13.

Lim, H. (2010) Effect of 'developmental speech and language training through music' on speech production children with autism spectrum disorders. *Journal of Music Therapy*, 47(1), 2–26.

Limb, C. J. (2008) Neural substrates of spontaneous musical performance: An fMRI study of jazz improvisation. *PLoS ONE*, 3(2). Retrieved from http://www.plosone.org/article/info%3Adoi%2F10.1371%2Fjournal.pone.0001679

Lin, Y., Dai, Y. and Hwang, S. (2003) The effect of reminiscence on the elderly population: A systematic review. *Public Health Nursing*, 20(4), 297–306.

Lincoln, Y. and Guba, E. (1985) *Naturalistic Inquiry*. Thousand Oaks, CA: Sage Publications.

Lincoln, Y. and Guba, E. (1986) But is it rigorous? Trustworthiness and authenticity in naturalistic evaluation. *New Directions for Program Evaluation, Special Issue: Naturalistic Evaluation*, 30, 73–84.

Lipgar, R. M. and Pines, M. (2003) *Building on Bion*. London: Jessica Kingsley.

Lipponen, A. (2005) Musiikki elvyttää vuorovaikutusta – kokemuksia musiikkiterapiasta päiväryhmässä. In S. Kalavainen (ed.) *Ensikodin Päiväryhmät: Kuvaus lastensuojelun vauvaperhetyön kehittymisestä*. Helsinki: Ensi-ja turvakotien liitto, pp. 107–19.

Lipponen, A. (2008) *Music Therapy for Early Interaction in High Risk Families: Learning, feeling and experiencing*. Paper presented at the Second International Music Therapy Research Conference, Laurier Centre for Music Therapy Research, Waterloo, Ontario.

Lipps, T. (1903) *Ästhetik: Psychologie des Schönen und der Kunst. Teil I. Grundlegung der Ästhetik*. Leipzig: Leopold Voss.

Loewy, J. (2000) Music psychotherapy assessment. *Music Therapy Perspectives*, 18, 47–58.

Loewy, J. V., Hallan, C., Friedman, E. and Martinez, C. (2005) Sleep/sedation in children undergoing EEG testing: A comparison of chloral hydrate and music therapy. *Journal of Perianaesthesia Nursing*, 20(5), 323–31.

Loewy, J. V. (2009) Musical sedation: Mechanisms of breathing entrainment. In R. Azoulay and J. V. Loewy (eds) *Music, the Breath, and Health: Advances in integrative music therapy*. New York: Satchnote Press, pp. 223–32.

Loganbill, C., Hardy, E. and Delworth, U. (1982) Supervision: A conceptual model. *The Counselling Psychologist*, 10(1), 3–42.

Lombardi, J. A., Surburg, P. and Koceja, D. (2000) Age differences and changes in midline-crossing inhibition in the lower extremities. *Journal of Gerontology: Medical Sciences*, 55A(5), M293–8.

López, V. (1970) *Acústica*. Madrid: Index.

Lozanov, G. (1971) *Suggestology and Outlines of Suggestopedy*. New York: Gordon and Breach.

Lysaker, P. H. and Lysaker, J. T. (2010) Schizophrenia and alterations in self-experience: A comparison of 6 perspectives. *Schizophrenia Bulletin*, 36(2), 331–40. doi: 10.1093/schbul/sbn077

Magee, W. L. and Burland, K. (2008) Using electronic music technologies in music therapy: Opportunities, limitations, and clinical indicators. *British Journal of Music Therapy*, 22(1), 3–15.

Magill, L. (2006) Music therapy and spirituality and the challenges of end-stage illness. In D. Aldridge and J. Fachner (eds) *Music and Altered States: Consciousness, transcendence, therapy, and addictions*. London: Jessica Kingsley, pp. 172–83.

Magne, C., Schön, D. and Besson, M. (2006) Musician children detect pitch violations in both music and language better than nonmusician children: Behavioural and electrophysical approaches. *Journal of Cognitive Neuroscience*, 18(199–211).

Mahler, M. S. (1975) *The Psychological Birth of the Human Infant*. New York: Basic Books.

Mahns, W. (1998) Symbol development in analytical music therapy with children: A qualitative study of the meaning of improvisation in music therapy with school children. Unpublished Dissertation. Aalborg University, Aalborg, Denmark.

Malloch, S. (1999) Mothers and infants and communicative musicality. In I. Deliège (ed.) *Rhythms, Musical Narrative, and the Origins of Human Communication*, Vol. Musicae Scientiae: Special Issue, 1999–2000, pp. 29–57. Liège: European Society for the Cognitive Sciences of Music.

Malloch, S. and Trevarthen, C. (2009) Communicative musicality: Exploring the basis of human companionship. Oxford: Oxford University Press.

Malterud, K. (2001a) The art and science of clinical knowledge: Evidence beyond measures and numbers. *The Lancet*, 358, 397–400.

Malterud, K. (2001b) Qualitative research: Standards, challenges, and guidelines. *The Lancet*, 358, 483–8.

Malyon, A. K. (1982) Psychotherapeutic implications of internalized homophobia in gay men. *Journal of Homosexuality*, 7(2–3), 59–69.

Mann, W. (1996) *Bottleneck Blues Guitar*. New York: Oak Publications.

Mannes, E. (2011) *The Power of Music: Pioneering discoveries in the new science of song*. New York: Walker & Company.

Marshak, M. (1960) A method for evaluating child–parent interactions under controlled conditions. *Journal of Genetic Psychology*, 97, 3–22.

Martin, D. J., Garske, J. P. and Davis, M. K. (2000) Relation of the therapeutic alliance with outcome and other variables: A meta-analytic review. *Journal of Counseling and Clinical Psychology*, 68(3), 438–50.

Martin, J. H. (1996) *Neuroanatomy: Textbook and atlas*. New York: McGraw Hill.

Martin, M. A. and Metha, A. (1997) Recall of early childhood memories through musical mood induction. *The Arts in Psychotherapy*, 24(5), 447–54.

Maslow, A. H. (1954) *Motivation and Personality*. New York: Harper.

Maslow, A. H. (1962) *Toward a Psychology of Being*. New York: Van Nostrand.

Maslow, A. H. (1964) *Religion, Values, and Peak Experiences*. New York: Viking.

Masserman, J. H. (1986) Poetry as music. *The Arts in Psychotherapy*, 13, 61–7.

Mateer, C. A. and Kerns, K. A. (2000) Capitalizing on neuroplasticity. *Cognition*, 41, 106–9.

Matell, M. S. and Meck, W. H. (2000) Neuropsychological mechanisms of interval timing behaviour. *BioEssays*, 22, 94–103.

Mays, N. and Pope, C. (1995) Rigour and qualitative research. *British Medical Journal*, 311, 109–12.

Mays, N. and Pope, C. (2000) Assessing quality in qualitative research. *British Medical Journal*, 320, 50–2.

McClary, R. (2007) Healing the psyche through music, myth, and ritual. *Psychology of Aesthetics, Creativity, and the Arts*, 1(3), 155–9.

McDonnell, L. (1983) Music therapy: Meeting the psychosocial needs of hospitalized children. *Journal of the Association for the Care of Children's Health*, 12(1), 29–33.

McFerrin, B. (1997) *Circlesongs* [CD]. New York: Sony Classical.

McGuire, M. G. (ed.) (2004) *Psychiatric Music Therapy in the Community: The legacy of Florence Tyson*. Gilsum, NH: Barcelona Publishers.

McKinney, J. R. and Thomas, R. E. (2010) Transference and countertransference. *Journal of Addictive Disorders*, 1–7.

McPherson, G. E. (ed.) (2006) *The Child as Musician: A handbook of musical development*. Oxford: Oxford University Press.

McWhirter, J. J., McWhirter, B. T., McWhirter, E. H. and McWhirter, R. J. (2007) *At-risk Youth: A comprehensive response for counselors, teachers, psychologists, and human service professionals.*, 4th edn. Belmont, CA: Thomson Higher Education.

Meltzer, F. (1990) Unconscious. In F. Lentricchia and T. McLaughlin (eds) *Critical Terms for Literary Study*. Chicago, IL: University of Chicago Press, pp. 147–62.

Menon, V. and Levitin, D. J. (2005) The rewards of music listening: Response and physiological connectivity of the mesolimbic system. *NeuroImage*, 28(1), 175–84.

Merrill, T. R. (2009) *The Music Therapy as Mentor: Two portraits of positive mentoring relationships*. East Lansing, MI: Michigan State University.

Meyer, K. (2011) Primary sensory cortices, top-down projections, and conscious experience. *Progress in Neurobiology*, 94(41), 408–17.

Meyer, P., De Villers, J. and Ebnet, E. (2010) *Guitar Skills for Music Therapists and Music Educators*. Gilsum, NH: Barcelona Publishers.

Michel, D. E. (1976) *Music Therapy: An introduction to therapy and special education through music*. Springfield, IL: Charles C. Thomas.

Michel, D. E. and Pinson, J. (2005) *Music Therapy in Principle and Practice*. Springfield, IL: Charles C. Thomas.

Micozzi, M. S. (2006) *Fundamentals of complementary and integrative medicine*, 3rd edn. St. Louis, MO: Saunders Elsevier.

Miller, E. B. (2011) *Bio-guided Music Therapy: A practitioner's guide to the clinical integration of music and biofeedback*. London: Jessica Kingsley.

Miller, J. J. (1999) The contributions of Wayne Ruppenthal to the field of music therapy. *Journal of Music Therapy*, 35(2), 105–18.

Miller, K. (1979) *Treatment with Music: A manual for allied health professionals*. Kalamazoo, MI: Department of Occupational Therapy, College of Health and Human Services, Michigan University.

Miller, M. C. (2009) Why does it feel good to improvise? *Harvard Mental Health Letter*, 25(9), 8.

Milton, M. and Coyle, A. (1999) Lesbian and gay affirmative psychotherapy: Issues in theory and practice. *Sexual and Marital Therapy*, 14(1), 43–59.

Mohanty, J. N. and McKenna, W. (eds) (1989) *Husserl's Phenomenology: A textbook*. Lanham, MD: University Press of America.

Montello, L. (1999) A psychoanalytic music therapy approach to treating adults traumatized as children. *Music Therapy Perspectives*, 17(2), 74–81.

Montgomery, C. (2002) Role of dynamic therapy in psychiatry. *Advances in Psychiatric*

Treatment, 8, 34–41.

Moore, B. E. and Fine, B. D. (1990) *Psychoanalytic Terms and Concepts*. New Haven, CT: The American Psychoanalytic Association and Yale University Press.

Moreira, S. V., França, C. C., Moreira, M. A. and Lana-Peixoto, M. A. (2009) Music identity of patients with multiple sclerosis. *Arquivos de Neuro-psiquiatria*, 67(1), 46–9.

Moreno, J. J. (1999) *Acting Your Inner Music: Music therapy and psychodrama*. Saint Louis, MO: MMB Music.

Moreno, J. J. (2006) *Acting Your Inner Music: Music therapy and psychodrama*, 2nd edn. Gilsum, NH: Barcelona Publishers.

Muchnik, S. (2006) *Genograms are a Useful Assessment Tool*. Paper presented at the American Counseling Association Convention.

Munro, S. (1984) *Music therapy in palliative/hospice care*. St Louis, MO: MMB.

Muran, J. C. and Barber, J. P. (2010) *The Therapeutic Alliance: An evidence-based guide to practice*. New York: Guilford Press.

Nachmanovitch, S. (1990) *Free Play: The power of improvisation in life and the arts*. New York: Jeremy P. Tarcher/Putnam.

Nakahara, H. (2009) Psycho-physiological responses to expressive piano performance. *International Journal of Psychophysiology*, 75, 268–76.

Naxos (2013a) A capella. *Naxos.com*. Retrieved from http://www.naxos.com/education/glossary.asp?char=A-C#

Naxos (2013b) Ostinato. Naxos.com. Retrieved from http://www.naxos.com/education/glossary.asp?char=M-O#

New York Times (1968, 18 March) Dr. Ira M. Altshuler, early user of music therapy, dies in crash, *The New York Times*, p. 45.

Newham, P. (1999) *Using Voice and Song in Therapy: The practical application of voice movement therapy*. London: Jessica Kingsley.

Nicholson, J. M., Berthelsen, D., Abad, V., Williams, K. and Bradley, J. (2008) Impact of music therapy to promote positive parenting and child development. *Journal of Health Psychology*, 13, 226–38.

Nocera, S. D. (1979) *Reaching the Special Learner Through Music*. Morristown, NJ: Silver Burdett.

Nolan, P. (1989a) Music as a transitional object in the treatment of bulimia. *Music Therapy Perspectives: Special Issue: The California Symposium on Clinical Practices*, 6, 49–51.

Nolan, P. (1989b) Music therapy improvisation techniques with bulimic patients. In K. Bruscia and L. M. Hornyak (eds) *Experiential Therapies for Eating Disorders*. New York: Guilford Press, pp. 167–90.

Nolte, J. (2008) *The Human Brain: An introduction to its functional anatomy*, 6th edn. New York: Mosby.

Nordoff, P. and Robbins, C. (1975) *Music Therapy in Special Education*. London: MacDonald & Evans.

Nordoff, P. and Robbins, C. (1977) *Creative Music Therapy: Individualized treatment for the handicapped child*. New York: John Day.

Nordoff, P. and Robbins, C. (2004) *Therapy in Music for Handicapped Children*. Gilsum, NH: Barcelona Publishers.

Nordoff, P. and Robbins, C. (2007) *Creative Music Therapy: A guide to fostering clinical musicianship*, 2nd edn. Gilsum, NH: Barcelona Publishers.

Nordoff, P., Robbins, C., Heyde, J., Levin, H. and Nowikas, S. (1995) *Greetings and Goodbyes*. Bryn Mawr, PA: Theodore Presser.

Nordoff, P. and Robbins, C. R. (1971) *Therapy in Music for Handicapped Children.* London: Gollancz.

Nordoff–Robbins Centre for Music Therapy (2013) Staff bios: Clive Robbins. Nordoff–Robbins Centre for Music Therapy, NYU Steinhardt School of Culture, Education and Human Development. Retrieved from http://steinhardt.nyu.edu/music/nordoff/staff#robbins

Norton, A., Zipse, L., Marchina, S. and Schlaug, G. (2009) Melodic intonation therapy: Shared insights on how it is done and why it might help. *Annals of the New York Academy of Sciences*, 1169, 431–6.

Novytskaya, L. (2009) *The infrasonic organization of the musical stream as the central part of the 'breathing' mechanism of the human brain.* Paper presented at the International Association for Music and Medicine Conference. Limerick, Ireland.

Noy, P. (1993) How music conveys emotion. In S. Feder, R. L. Karmel and G. Pollock (eds) *Psychoanalytic Explorations in Music. Second series.* Madison, CT: International Universities Press.

Nygaard Pederson, I. (1999) Music therapy as holding and re-organizing work with schizophrenic and psychotic patients. In T. Wigram and J. De Backer (eds) *Clinical Applications of Music Therapy in Psychiatry*. London: Jessica Kingsley, pp. 24–43.

Odell-Miller, H. and Richards, E. (2009) *Supervision of Music Therapy: A theoretical and practical handbook.* London: Routledge.

Ogletree, E. J. (1976) Eurythmy: A therapeutic art of movement. *The Journal of Special Education*, 10(3), 305–19.

O'Gorman, S. (2006) Theoretical interfaces in the acute paediatric context: A psychotherapeutic understanding of the application of infant-directed singing. *American Journal of Psychotherapy*, 60(3), 271–83.

Oldfield, A. (2006a) *Interactive Music Therapy: A positive approach.* London: Jessica Kingsley Publishers.

Oldfield, A. (2006b) *Interactive Music Therapy in Child and Family Psychiatry: Clinical practical, research, and teaching.* London: Jessica Kingsley.

Oldfield, A. and Flower, C. (eds) (2008) *Music Therapy with Children and their Families.* London: Jessica Kingsley.

Omaha, J. (2004) *Psychotherapeutic Interventions for Emotion Regulation: EMDR and bilateral stimulation for affect management.* New York: Norton.

O'Reilly, A.-M. (2008) Music therapy. St Joseph's Foundation. Retrieved from www.stjosephsfoundation.ie/musictheropy2008–003.htm

Orff, C. (1994) The Schulwerk and music therapy: Carl Off, 1964. *The Orff Echo*, 26(4), 10–13.

Orff, G. (1980) *Orff music Therapy: Active furthering of the development of the child.* St Louis, MO: MMB Music.

Orff, G. (1989) *Key concepts in the Orff Music Therapy*, translated by J. Day and S. Salmon. London: Scott & Co.

Osborne, N. (2009) Towards a chronobiology of musical rhythm. In S. Malloch and C. Trevarthen (eds) *Communicative Musicality: Exploring the basis of human companionship*. Oxford: Oxford University Press, pp. 545–64.

Paipare, M. (2011) Music therapy. In R. Märtinsone (ed.) *Art Therapy*. Riga, Latvia: Raka.

Palmer, C. and Hutchins, S. (2006) What is musical prosody? In B. H. Ross (ed.) *The Psychology of Learning and Motivation: Advances in research and theory*, 46, 245–62. Amsterdam: Elsevier.

Panksepp, J. and Bernatzky, G. (2002) Emotional sounds and the brain: The neuroaffective foundations of musical appreciation. *Behavioral Processes*, 60, 133–55.

Pasiali, V. (2010) *Family-based Music Therapy: Fostering child resilience and promoting parental self-efficacy through shared musical experiences.* (Unpublished doctoral dissertation). Michigan State University, East Lansing, MI. Retrieved from http://search.proquest.com/docview/746773159?accountid=38688

Patel, A. D. (2008) *Music, Language, and the Brain*. Oxford: Oxford University Press.

Patton, M. (1999) Enhancing the quality and credibility of qualitative analysis. *Health Services*

Pavlicevic, M. (1997) *Music Therapy in Context: Music, meaning and relationship.* London: Jessica Kingsley.

Pavlicevic, M. (2003) *Groups in Music: Strategies from music therapy*. London: Jessica Kingsley.

Pavlicevic, M. and Ansdell, G. (eds) (2004) *Community Music Therapy*. London: Jessica Kingsley.

Pavlicevic, M., Trevarthen, C. and Duncan, J. (1994) Improvisational music therapy and the rehabilitation of persons suffering from chronic schizophrenia. *Journal of Music Therapy*, 31(2), 88–104.

Pedersen, I. N. (2007) Countertransference in music therapy. Unpublished PhD Dissertation. Aalborg University, Aalborg, Denmark.

Peretz, I. (2006) The nature of music from a biological perspective. *Cognition*, 100(1), 1–32.

Peters, J. (1987) *Music Therapy: An introduction*. Springfield, IL: Charles C. Thomas.

Platel, H. (2005) Functional neuroimaging of semantic and episodic musical memory. *Annals of the New York Academy of Sciences*, 1060, 136–47.

Pollard, J. (2004) We must stop meeting like this. In M. Luca (ed.) *The Therapeutic Frame in the Clinical Context: Integrative perspectives*. Hove and New York: Brunner-Routledge, pp. 98–115.

Popay, J., Roberts, H., Sowden, A., Petticrew, M., Arai, L., Rodgers, M., Britten, N., Roen K. and Duffy, S. (2006) *Guidance on the Conduct of Narrative Synthesis in Systematic Reviews.* Economic and Social Research Council Methods Programme.

Porchet-Munro, S. (1993) Music therapy perspectives in palliative care education. *Journal of Palliative Care*, 9(4), 39–42.

Portnoy, J. (1963) *Music in the Life of Man*. New York: Holt, Rinehart and Winston.

Pratt, R. R. and Spintge, R. R. (1995) *MusicMedicine*, 2. Saint Louis, MO: MMB.

Price, R. H. and Lorion, R. P. (1989) Prevention programming as organizational reinvention: From research to implementation. In D. Shaffer, I. Philips and N. B. Enzer (eds) *Prevention of Mental Disorders, Alcohol and Other Drug Use in Children and Adolescents*. Rockville, MD: US Department of Health and Human Services, pp. 97–123.

Priestley, M. (1975) *Music Therapy in Action*, 2nd edn. St Louis, MO: MMB Music.

Priestley, M. (1994) *Essays on Analytical Music Therapy*. Gilsum, NH: Barcelona Publishers.

Priestley, M. and Eschen, J. T. (2002) Analytical music therapy: Origin and development. In J. T. Eschen (ed.) *Analytical Music Therapy*. London: Jessica Kingsley, pp. 74–87.

Procter, S. (2002) Empowering and enabling: Music therapy in non-medical mental health provision. In C. Kenny and B. Stige (eds) *Contemporary Voices in Music Therapy*. Oslo: Unipub Forlag, pp. 95–108.

Quintana, M., Storck, N., Lindblad, L. E., Lindvall, K. and Ericson, M. (1997) Heart rate variability as a means of assessing prognosis after acute myocardial infarction: A 3-year follow-up study. *European Heart Journal*, 5, 789–97.

Radstone, S. and Hodgkin, K. (eds) (2003) *Regimes of Memory*. London: Routledge.

Randel, D. M. (ed.) (2003) Cambridge, MA: Belknap Press of Harvard University.

Ratner, L. G. (1966) *Music: The listener's art*. New York: McGraw-Hill.

Reason, P. and Bradbury, H. (2006) *The Handbook of Action Research*. London: Sage Publications.

Reimer, B. (1970) *A Philosophy of Music Education*. Englewood Cliffs, CA: Prentice-Hall.

Reiter, S. (ed.) (2009) *Writing Away the Demons: Stories of creative coping through transformative writing*. St Cloud, MN: North Star Press.

Richards, P. R. (2010) Everyday creativity: Process and way of life – four key issues. In J. C. Kaufman and R. J. Sternberg (eds) *The Cambridge Handbook of Creativity*. New York: Cambridge University Press, pp. 189–215.

Ricoeur, P. (1978) *The Rule of Metaphor: Multi-disciplinary studies of the creation of meaning in language*. London: Routledge.

Ridder, H. M., Wigram, T. and Ottesen, A. M. (2009) A pilot study on the effects of music therapy on frontotemporal dementia: developing a research protocol. *Nordic Journal of Music Therapy*, 18(2), 103–32.

Rider, M. (1997) *The Rhythmic Language of Health and Disease*. Saint Louis, MO: MMB Music.

Rider, M. (1999) Homeodynamic mechanisms of improvisational music therapy. In C. Dileo (ed.) *Music Therapy and Medicine: Theoretical and clinical applications*. Silver Spring, MD: AMTA, pp. 107–14.

Riganello, F., Candelieri, A., Quintieri, M. and Dolce, G. (2010) Heart rate variability, emotions, and music. *Journal of Psychophysiology*, 24(2), 112–19.

Rio, R. (2002) Improvisation with the elderly: Moving from creative activities to process-oriented therapy. *The Arts in Psychotherapy*, 29, 191–201.

Ritholz, M. and Robbins, C. (1999) *Themes for Therapy from the Nordoff–Robbins Music Therapy Center at New York University*. New York: Carl Fischer.

Ritholz, M. and Robbins, C. (2003) *More Themes for Therapy from the Nordoff–Robbins Music Therapy Center at New York University*. New York: Carl Fischer.

Rizzolatti, G. and Sinigaglia, C. (2008) *Mirrors in the Brain: How our minds share actions, emotions, and experience*. New York: Oxford University Press.

Robb, S. L. (2000) Music assisted progressive muscle relaxation, progressive muscle relaxation, music listening, and silence: A comparison of relaxation techniques *Journal of Music Therapy*, 37(1), 2–21.

Robbins, C. (1997) *What a Wonderful Song Her Life Sang: An anthology of appreciation for Carol Robbins*. New York: The International Trust for Nordoff–Robbins Music Therapy.

Robbins, C. (2005) *A journey into Creative Music Therapy*, 3. St Louis, MO: MMB Music.

Robbins, C. and Forinash, M. (1991) A time paradigm: Time as a multilevel phenomenon in music therapy. *Music Therapy*, 10, 46–57.

Robbins, C. and Robbins, C. (1980) *Music for the Hearing Impaired and Other Special Groups*. St Louis, MO: MMB Music.

Robbins, C. and Robbins, C. (1991a) Self-communications in Creative Music Therapy. In K. E. Bruscia (ed.) *Case Studies in Music Therapy*. Gilsum, NH: Barcelona Publishers, pp. 55–72.

Robbins, C. and Robbins, C. (1991b) Creative Music Therapy in bringing order, change and communicativeness to the life of a brain-injured adolescent. In K. E. Bruscia (ed.) *Case Studies in Music Therapy*. Gilsum, NH: Barcelona Publishers, pp. 231–49.

Robbins, C. and Robbins, C. (1998) *Healing Heritage: Paul Nordoff exploring the tonal language of music.* Gilsum, NH: Barcelona Publishers.

Roberts, A. (2008, 27 April) First person action research. *Andy Roberts DARnet.* Retrieved from http://distributedresearch.net/blog/2008/04/27/first-person-action-research

Roberts, R. (2003) *Voices of Authenticity and Integrity: A music therapist's self-inquiry in working with children facing life-threatening illness.* (Unpublished Masters dissertation). Wilfrid Laurier University, Waterloo, Ontario.

Rock, A., Trainor, L. J. and Addison, T. (1999) Distinctive messages in infant-directed lullabies and play songs. *Developmental Psychology*, 35(2), 527–34.

Roehrborn, H. (2007) Dyadic regulative music therapy: Experiences from a psychotherapy ward of a hospital. In I. Frohne-Hagemann (ed.) *Receptive Music Therapy: theory and practice.* Wiesbaden: Reichert Verlag, pp. 211–22.

Rogers, C. (1951) *Client-centered Therapy: Its current practice, implications and theory.* London: Constable.

Rogers, C. (1954) Becoming a person: A lecture delivered on the Nellie Heldt Lecture Fund. Chicago, IL: University of Chicago.

Rogers, C. (1959) A theory of therapy, personality and interpersonal relationships as developed in the client-centered framework. In S. Koch (ed.) *Formulations of the Person and the Social Context*, 3. New York: McGraw Hill.

Rogers, C. (1961) *On Becoming a Person: A therapist's view of psychotherapy.* London: Constable.

Rogers, C. (1980) *A Way of Being.* Boston: Houghton Mifflin.

Rojo, N., Amengual, J., Juncadella, M., Robio, F., Camara, E., Marco-Pallares, J. and Rodriguez-Fornells, A. (2011) Music-Supported Therapy induces plasticity in the sensorimotor cortex in chronic stroke: A single-case study using multimodal imaging (fMRI-TMS). *Brain Injury*, 25, 787–93. doi: 10.3109/02699052.2011.576305

Rolvsjord, R. (2010) *Resource-oriented Music Therapy in Mental Health Care.* Gilsum, NH: Barcelona Publishers.

Rosen, H. (1998) *Speaking from Memory: A guide to autobiographical acts and practices.* Oakhill: Trentham Books.

Rouget, G. (1985) *Music and Trance: A theory of the relations between music and possession.* Chicago, IL: University of Chicago Press.

Rubin, J. A. (2001) *Approaches to Art Therapy.* Philadelphia, PA: Brunner and Mazel.

Russo, R., Whittuck, D., Roberson, D., Dutton, K., Georgiou, G. and Fox, E. (2006) Mood-congruent free recall bias in anxious individuals is not a consequence of response bias. *Memory*, 14(4), 393–9. doi: 10.1080/09658210500343166

Rust, P. C. (2003) Finding a sexual identity and community: Therapeutic implications and cultural assumptions in scientific models of coming out. In L. D. Garnets and D. C. Kimmel (eds) *Psychological Perspectives on Lesbian, Gay, and Bisexual Experiences*, 2nd edn. New York: Columbia University Press Books, pp. 227–69.

Ruud, E. (1980) *Music Therapy and its Relationship to Current Treatment Theories.* St Louis, MO: Magna Music Baton.

Ruud, E. (1988) Music therapy: Health profession or cultural movement? *Music Therapy*, 7(1), 34–7.

Ruud, E. (1997) Music and identity. *Norsk Tidsskrift for Musikkterapi*, 6(1), 3–13.

Ruud, E. (1998) *Music Therapy: Improvisation, communication, and culture.* Gilsum, NH: Barcelona Publishers.

Ruud, E. (2010) *Music Therapy: A perspective from the humanities.* Gilsum, NH:

Barcelona Publishers.

Safran, J. D., Muran, J. C., Samstag, L. and Winston, A. (2005) Evaluating alliance-focused intervention for potential treatment failures. *Psychotherapy*, 42, 532–45.

Salimpoor, V. N., Benovoy, M., Larcher, K., Dagher, A. and Zatorre, R. J. (2011) Anatomically distinct dopamine release during anticipation and experience of peak emotion to music. *Nature Neuroscience*, 14(2), 257–62.

Sanville, J. B. (1999) Meaning making and playing in psychoanalytic therapies. *Smith College Studies in Social Work*, 69(3), 509–23.

Särkämö, T., Tervaniemi, M., Laitinen, S., Forsblom, A., Soinila, S., Mikkonen, M. and Hietanen, M. (2008) Music listening enhances cognitive recovery and mood after middle cerebral artery stroke. *Brain*, 131, 866–76.

Särkämö, T., Pihko, E., Laitinen, S., Soinila, S., Mikkonen, M. and Tervaniemi, M. (2010) Music and speech listening enhance the recovery of early sensory processing after stroke. *Journal of Cognitive Neuroscience*, 22, 2716–27. doi: 10.1162/jocn.2009.21376

Saxon, W. (2001, January 31) Florence Tyson, 82, early advocate of creative arts therapy [Obituary]. *New York Times*. Retrieved from http://www.nytimes.com/2001/01/31/nyregion/florence-tyson-82-early-advocate-of-creative-arts-therapy.html

Schauer, M. and Mauritz, K. (2003) Musical motor feedback (MMF) in walking hemi-paretic stroke patients: Randomized trials of gait improvement. *Clinical Rehabilitation*, 17(1), 713–22. doi: 10.1191/0269215503cr668oa

Scheiby, B. B. (1998) Listen to the music of the unconscious: Using countertransference as a compass in analytical music therapy. In A. Robbins (ed.) *Therapeutic Presence*. London: Jessica Kingsley, pp. 185–203.

Scheiby, B. B. (2005) An intersubjective approach to music therapy: identification and processing of musical countertransference in a music psychotherapeutic context. In *Music Therapy Perspectives*, 23, 8–17.

Scheiby, B. B. (2013) Analytical Music Therapy, Priestley Method. In Wheeler, B.L. (ed.) *Music Therapy Handbook*. New York: Guildford Press.

Scheiby, B.B. and Pedersen, I. N. (1999) Inter music therapy in the training of music therapy students. *Nordic Journal of Music Therapy*, 8(1). p58–71.

Schiff, A. W. and Schiff, J. L. (1971) Passivity. *Transactional Analysis Journal*, 1(1), 71–8.

Schmid, W. and Ostermann, T. (2010) Home-based music therapy: A systematic overview of settings and conditions for an innovative service in healthcare. *BMC Health Services Research*, 10(291), 1–10. doi: 10.1186/1472-6963-10-291

Schmidt-Jones, C. (2011) Vocables: Easy vocal improvisation activities. *Connexions*. Retrieved from http://cnx.org/content/m17623/latest/

Schneck, D. J. and Berger, D. S. (2006) *The Music Effect: Music physiology and clinical applications*. London: Jessica Kingsley Publishers.

Schneider, S., Münte, T. F., Rodriguez-Fornells, A., Sailer, M. and Altemüller, E. (2010) Music supported training is more efficient than functional motor training for recovery of fine motor skills in stroke patients. *Music Perception*, 27(4), 271–80.

Schneider, S., Schönle, P. W., Altemüller, E. and Münte, T. F. (2007) Using musical instruments to improve motor skill recovery following a stroke. *Journal of Neurology*, 254(10), 1339–46.

Schulberg, C. (1981) *The Music Therapy Sourcebook*. New York: Human Sciences Press.

Schumacher, K. (1999) *Musiktherapie und Såulingsforschung*. Frankfurt: Peter Lang.

Schwabe, C. (2007) Regulatory Music Therapy (RMT): Milestones of a conceptual development. In I. Frohne-Hagemann (ed.) *Receptive Music Therapy and Practice*. Wiesbaden: Reichert Verlag, pp. 203–10.

Scovel, M. A. and Gardstrom, S. C. (2002) Music therapy within the context of psychotherapeutic models. In R. F. Unkefer and M. H. Thaut (eds) *Music Therapy in the Treatment of Adults with Mental Disorders: Theatrical bases and clinical information*, 2nd edn. St Louis: MMB Music, pp. 117–32.

Sears, M. S. (ed.) (2007) *Music: The therapeutic edge: Readings from William S. Sears*. Gilsum, NH: Barcelona Publishers.

Sears, W. W. (1968) Processes in music therapy. In E. T. Gaston (ed.) *Music Therapy*. New York: MacMillan, pp. 30–44.

Sewell, W. H. (1992) A theory of structure: Duality, agency, and transformation. *American Journal of Sociology*, 98(1), 1–29.

Sharp, D., Snyder, R. and Hischke, J. (1998) *An Outline History of American Jazz*. Dubuque, IA: Kendall/Hunt Publishing.

Sharpe, N. (1977) The history of the CAMT. *The Journal: CAMT*, 5(2), 2.

Shaw, A. (1986) *Black Popular Music in America: The singers, songwriters, and musicians who pioneered the sounds of American music*. New York: Schirmer Books.

Shebib, B. (2003) *Choices: Interviewing and counseling skills for Canadians*, 2nd edn. Toronto, ON: Pearson.

Sherratt, K., Thornton, A. and Hatton, C. (2004) Music interventions for people with dementia: A review of the literature. *Aging and Mental Health*, 8(1), 3–12.

Sherrington, C. S. (1906) *The Integrative Action of the Nervous System*. New York: Charles Scribner's Sons.

Shields, A. and Robbins, A. (1980) Music in expressive therapy. In A. Robbins (ed.) *Expressive Therapy: A creative arts approach to depth-oriented treatment*. New York: Human Sciences Press, pp. 239–57.

Shoemark, H. and Grocke, D. E. (2010) The markers of interplay between the music therapist and the medically fragile newborn infant. *Journal of Music Therapy*, 47, 306–34.

Shugar, B. (2009) An interview with Susan Munro-Porchet. *Voices: A world forum for music therapy*, 9(3). Retrieved from https://normt.uib.no/index.php/voices/article/viewArticle/334/260

Shushardzhan, S. (1994) *Health on the Notes: Workshop path to spiritual perfection and waking longevity*. Moscow: izd-vo AO 'Perspective'.

Shushardzhan, S. (1995) Experiences of using vocal therapy in a clinic for internal illnesses. *Medical Technologies*, 1–2, 62–3.

Shushardzhan, S. (1999) *Psychophysiological and Biophysical Bases of Music and Vocal Therapy Adaptive and Reviving Effects*. (Unpublished doctoral dissertation). Sechenov Moscow Medical Academy, Moscow.

Shushardzhan, S. (2001) *Music Acupuncture Therapy as a Method of Psychosomatic Correction*. Paper presented at the Zdravnitsa 2001. Moscow: Ministry of Health and Social Development of the Russian Federation.

Shushardzhan, S., Shushardzhan, R. and Eremina, N. (2008) Traditional conception of music therapy and reflex-resonant theory of musical-acoustic influences. *Traditional Medicine*, 2(13), 32–7.

Shuter-Dyson, R. (1982) Musical ability. In D. Deutsch (ed.) *The Psychology of Music*. New York: Academic Press, pp. 391–412.

Siegel, D. (2001) Toward an interpersonal neurobiology of the developing mind:

Attachment relationships, 'mindsight', and neural integration. *Infant Mental Health Journal*, 22(1–2), 67–94.

Siegelman, E. (1990) *Metaphor and Meaning in Psychotherapy*. New York: Guildford Press.

Shebib, B. (2003) *Choices: Interviewing and counseling skills for Canadians*, 2nd edn. Toronto, ON: Pearson.

Silverman, M. (2007) The effect of paired pitch, rhythm, and speech on working memory as measured by sequential digit recall. *Journal of Music Therapy*, 44(4), 415–27.

Silvermann, Y. (2004) The story within: Myth and fairy tale in therapy. *The Arts in Psychotherapy*, 31, 127–35.

Skille, O. and Wigram, T. (1995) The effect of music, vocalization, and vibration on brain and muscle tissues: Studies in vibroacoustic therapy. In T. Wigram, B. Saperston and R. West (eds) *The Art and Science of Music Therapy: A handbook*. New York: Routledge, pp. 23–57.

Skille, O. (1997) Making music for vibroacoustic therapy. In T. Wigram and C. Dileo (eds) *Music, Vibration, and Health*. Cherry Hill, NJ: Jeffrey Books, pp. 235–4.

Slavson, S. R. and Schiffer, M. (1975) *Group Psychotherapies for Children: A textbook*. New York: International Universities Press.

Sloboda, J. (1985) *The Musical Mind: The cognitive psychology of music*. Oxford: Clarendon Press.

Sloboda, J. (2005) *Exploring the Musical Mind*. Oxford: Oxford University Press.

Sloboda, J. A. (1991) Musical structure and emotional response: Sound empirical findings. *Psychology of Music*, 19, 110–20.

Small, C. (1998) *Musicking: The meanings of performing and listening*. Hanover: University Press of New England.

Smeijsters, H. (1993) Music therapy and psychotherapy. *The Arts in Psychotherapy*, 20, 223–9.

Smeijsters, H. (2005a) Quantitative single case designs. In B. L. Wheeler (ed.) *Music Therapy Research*, 2nd edn. Phoenixville, PA: Barcelona Publishers, pp. 293–305.

Smeijsters, H. (2005b) *Sounding the Self: Analogy in improvisational music therapy*. Gilsum, NH: Barcelona Publishers.

Smeijsters, H. (2006) Research in practice. *Music Therapy Today*, 7(4), 781–838.

Somody, C. (2010) *Meaning and Connections in Older Populations: A phenomenological study of reminiscence using a musical chronology and the emerging life song*. (Unpublished doctoral dissertation). University of Texas, San Antonio. (UMI 3433230).

Southern, E. (1997) *The Music of Black Americans: A history*, 3rd edn. New York: W. W. Norton Publishing.

Sorel, S. (2011) *Writing Humanistic Music Therapy Goal in an Evidence-based World*. Paper presented at the American Music Therapy Association, Atlanta, Georgia.

Soria-Urios, G., Duque, P. and García-Moreno, J. M. (2011) Música y cerebro: fundamentos neurocientíficos y trastornos musicales. *Revista de Neurologia*, 52, 45–55.

Sparks, R. W., Helm, N. A. and Albert, M. L. (1973) Melodic intonation therapy for aphasia. *Archives of Neurology*, 29, 130–1.

Sparks, R. W. and Deck, J. W. (1986) Melodic intonation therapy. In R. Chipley (ed.) *Language Intervention Strategies in Adult Aphasia*. Baltimore, MD: Williams and Wilkins.

Spence, M. J. and DeCasper, A. J. (1987) Prenatal experience with low frequency maternal-voice sounds influence neonatal perception of maternal voice samples. *Infant Behavior and Development*, 10, 133–42.

Spencer, L., Ritchie, J., Lewis, J. and Dillon, L. (2003) *Quality in Qualitative Evaluation: A framework for assessing research evidence*. London: Government Chief Social Researcher's Office, UK.

Spintge, R. R. and Droh, R. (1987) *Music in Medicine*. Heidelberg and New York: Springer.

Spintge, R. R. and Droh, R. (1993) *MusicMedicine*. Saint Louis, MO: MMB.

Stake, R. (1995) *The Art of Case Study Research*. Thousand Oaks, CA: Sage Publications.

Steele, P. (1984) Aspects of resistance in music therapy: Theory and technique. *Music Therapy*, 4(1), 64–72.

Stein, D. G. (2000) Brain injury and theories of recovery. In A. L. Christensen and B. P. Uzzell (eds) *International Handbook of Neuropsychological Rehabilitation: Critical issues in neuropsychology* (pp. 9–32). New York: Kluwer Academic/Plenum Publishers.

Stein, R. (1991) *Psychoanalytic Theories of Affect*. London: Karnac Books.

Steiner, R. (1983) *The Inner Nature of Music and the Experience of Tone: Selected lectures from the work of Rudolf Steiner (GA 283)*. London: Rudolf Steiner Press.

Stern, D. N. (1977) *The First Relationship: Infant and mother*. London: Open Books.

Stern, D. N. (1985a) *The Interpersonal World of the Infant: A view from psychoanalysis and developmental psychology*. New York: Basic Books.

Stern, D. N. (1985b) Affect attunement. In J. D. Call, E. Galenson and R. L. Tyson (eds) *Frontiers of infant psychiatry*, 2. New York: Basic Books.

Stern, D. N. (2010) *Forms of Vitality*. Oxford: Oxford University Press.

Stevens, M. J. and Morris, S. J. (1995) A format for case conceptualization. *Counselor Education and Supervision*, 35, 82–94.

Stewart, K. and Schneider, S. (2000) The effects of music therapy on the sound environment in the NICU: A pilot study. In J. V. Loewy (ed.) *Music Therapy in the Neonatal Intensive Care Unit*. New York: Satchnote Press, pp. 85–100.

Stige, B. (2002a) *Culture-centered Music Therapy*. Gilsum, NH: Barcelona Publishers.

Stige, B. (2002b) The relentless roots of music therapy. *Voices: A world forum for music therapy*, 2(3). Retrieved from https://normt.uib.no/index.php/voices/article/viewArticle/98/75

Stige, B. (2003) *Elaborations Toward a Notion of Community Music Therapy*. Oslo: Unipub.

Stige, B. (2005) Participatory action research. In B. L. Wheeler (ed.) *Music Therapy Research*. Gilsum, NH: Barcelona Publishers, pp. 404–15.

Stige, B. (2006) Toward a notion of participation in music therapy. *Nordic Journal of Music Therapy*, 15(2), 121–38.

Stige, B. (2010) Musical participation, social space, and everyday ritual. In B. Stige, G. Ansdell, C. Elefant and M. Pavlicevic (eds) *Where Music Helps: Community music therapy in action and reflection*. Aldershot: Ashgate Publishing.

Stige, B. (2012) Health Musicking: A Perspective on Music and Health as Action and Performance. In MacDonald, R., Kreutz, G. and Mitchell, L. (eds). *Music, Health and Wellbeing*. Oxford: Oxford University Press, 183–95.

Stige, B. and Aarø, L. E. (2012) *Invitation to Community Music Therapy*. New York: Routledge.

Stige, B., Malterud, K. and Midtgarden, T. (2009) Toward an agenda for evaluation of qualitative research. *Qualitative Health Research*, 19(10), 1504–16.

Strickland, E. (2011) Beat: The seventh sense. *Discover Magazine Presents the Brain*, Spring, 12–16.

Storr, A. (1992) *Music and the Mind.* New York: Ballantine Books.

Summer, L. (2002) Group music and imagery therapy: Emergent receptive techniques in music therapy practice. In K. Bruscia and D. E. Grocke (eds) *Guided Imagery and Music: The Bonny method and beyond.* Gilsum, NH: Barcelona Publishers, pp. 297–306.

Summers, R. F. and Barber, J. P. (2003) Therapeutic alliance as a measurable psychotherapy skill. *Academic Psychiatry*, 27(3). doi: 10.1176/appi.ap.27.3.160

Summers, S. (1999) *A Tapestry of Voices: Community building with a geriatric choir.* (Unpublished master's thesis). British Columbia Open University, Burnaby, BC.

Summers, S. (2011) The vocal *Hello Space* model in hospice music therapy. In F. A. Baker and S. Uhlig (eds) *Voicework in Music Therapy*. London: Jessica Kingsley, pp. 302–20.

Taetle, L. and Cutietta, R. (2002) Learning theories as roots of current musical practice and research. In R. Colwell and C. Richardson (eds) *The New Handbook of Research on Music Teaching and Learning: A project of the music educators national conference.* New York: Oxford University Press, pp. 279–98.

Tamplin, J. (2006) Song collage technique: A new approach to songwriting. *Nordic Journal of Music Therapy*, 15, 177–91.

Tan, S.-L., Pfordresher, P. and Harré, R. (2010) *Psychology of Music: From sound to significance.* Hove and New York: Psychology Press.

Tanner, D. R. and O'Bright, R. M. (1980) Music can color a graying America. *Music Educators Journal*, 67, 28–30.

Tart, C. (1972) States of consciousness and state-specific sciences. *Science*, 175, 1203–10.

Tashakkori, A. and Teddlie, C. (eds) (2010) *Sage Handbook of Mixed Methods in Social and Behavioral Research*, 2nd edn. Thousand Oaks, CA: Sage Publications.

Taylor, D. B. (1997) *Biomedical Foundations of Music Therapy.* Saint Louis, MO: MMB Music.

Taylor, E. (1998) The theory and practice of transformative learning: A critical review. In Center on Education and Training for Employment, College of Education (Information Series no. 374). Columbus, OH: ERIC Clearinghouse of adult, career, and vocational edition.

Telegraph (2012, 18 January) Clive Robbins [Obituary]. *The Telegraph.* Retrieved from http://www.telegraph.co.uk/news/obituaries/9023645/Clive-Robbins.html

Tervo, J. (2005) Music therapy with adolescents. *Voices: A World Forum for Music Therapy*, 5(1). Retrieved from https://normt.uib.no/index.php/voices/article/view/216/160

Thane, E. (2011) Vocal-led relaxation for children with autism spectrum disorders. In F. A. Baker and S. Uhlig (eds) *Voicework in Music Therapy*. London: Jessica Kingsley, pp. 41–62.

Thaut, M. H. (2005) *Rhythm, Music, and the Brain: Scientific foundations and clinical applications.* New York: Routledge.

Thaut, M. H., Mertel, K. and Leins, A. K. (2008) Music therapy for children and adults with physical disabilities. In W. B. Davis, K. E. Gfeller and M. H. Thaut (eds) *An Introduction to Music Therapy: Theory and practice*, 3rd edn. Silver Spring, MD: American Music Therapy Association, pp. 143–80.

Thaut, M. H., Thaut, C. and LaGasse, B. (2008) Music therapy in neurologic rehabilitation. In W. B. Davis, K. E. Gfeller and M. H. Thaut (eds) *An introduction to music therapy: Theory and practice*, 3rd edn. Silver Spring, MD: American Music Therapy Association, pp. 261–304.

Thompson, W. F., Schellenberg, E. G. and Husain, G. (2003) Perceiving prosody in speech: Effects of music lessons. *Annals of the New York Academy of Sciences*, 999, 530–32.

Thompson, W. F., Schellenberg, E. G. and Husain, G. (2004) Decoding speech prosody: Do music lessons help? *Emotion*, 4, 46–64.

Tomaino, C. M. (2009) Clinical applications of music therapy in neurologic rehabilitation. In R. Haas and V. Brandes (eds) *Music That Works: Contributions of biology, neurophysiology, psychology, sociology, medicine, and musicology*. Vienna: Springer, pp. 211–20.

Tong, A., Sainsbury, P. and Craig, J. (2007) Consolidated criteria for reporting qualitative research (COREQ): A 32-item checklist for interviews and focus groups. *International Journal for Quality in Health Care*, 9(6), 349–57.

Towse, E. (1997) Group analysis and improvisation: A musical perspective. *British Journal of Music Therapy*, 11(2), 51–5.

Trainor, L. J., Austin, C. and Desjardins, R. (2000) Is infant-directed speech prosody a result of the vocal expression of emotion? *Psychological Science*, 11(3), 188–95.

Travis, F. and Pearson, C. (1999) Pure consciousness: Distinct phenomenological and physiological correlates of 'consciousness itself'. *International Journal of Neuroscience*, 100, 77–89.

Trehub, S. (1990) The perception of musical patterns by human infants: The provision of similar patterns by their parents. In M. A. Berkley and W. C. Stebbins (eds) *Comparative perception* (Vol. 1: *Mechanisms*, pp. 429–59). New York: Wiley.

Trehub, S. and Schellenberg, E. G. (1995) Music: Its relevance to infants. *Annals of Child Development*, 11, 1–24.

Trehub, S., Unyk, A. and Trainor, L. J. (1993) Maternal singing in cross-cultural perspective. *Infant Behaviour and Development*, 16, 285–95.

Trevarthen, C. (1999) Musicality and the intrinsic motive pulse: Evidence from human psychobiology and infant communication. In I. Deliège (ed.) *Rhythms, Musical Narrative, and the Origins of Human Communication* (Vol. *Musicae Scientiae: Special Issue, 1999–2000*, pp. 157–213). Liège: European Society for the Cognitive Sciences of Music.

Trevarthen, C. (2008) The musical art of infant conversation: Narrating in the time of sympathetic experience, without rational interpretation, before words *Narrative in Music and Interaction* (Vol. *Musicae Scientiae: Special Issue*, 20 March 2008, pp. 15–46). Liège: European Society for the Cognitive Sciences of Music.

Trevarthen, C. (2009) Human biochronology: On the source and function of musicality. In R. Haas and V. Brandes (eds) *Music That Works: Contributions of biology, neurophysiology, psychology, sociology, medicine, and musicology*. Vienna and New York: Springer, pp. 221–66.

Trevarthen, C. and Malloch, S. N. (2000) The dance of wellbeing: Defining the musical therapeutic effect. *Nordic Journal of Music Therapy*, 9(2), 3–17.

Trondalen, G. (2002) En fenomenologisk inspirert arbeidsprosedyre for analyse av improvisasjoner i musikkterapeutisk praksis: Et narrativt perspektiv. In E. Nesheim, I. M. Hanken and B. Bjøtegaard (eds) *Flerstemmige inspill*, 2, 51–74. Oslo: NMH-publikasjoner.

Tronick, E. (1998) Dyadically expanded states of consciousness and the process of therapeutic change. *Infant Mental Health Journal*, 19(3), 290–99.

Tucker, J. (2005) *Multidimensional Music Therapy*. Victoria, BC: Trafford Publishing.

Tyson, E. (2002) Hip hop therapy: An exploratory study of a rap music intervention with at-risk and delinquent youth. *Journal of Poetry Therapy*, 15(3), 131–44.

Uhlig, S. and Baker, F. A. (2011) Voicework in music therapy: Pioneers and a new generation. In F. A. Baker and S. Uhlig (eds) *Voicework in Music Therapy: Research and practice*. London: Jessica Kingsley, pp. 25–42.

United States Department of Health and Human Services (2010) *Focus on Prevention*. Publication No. (SMA) 10–4120. Rockville, MD: Center for Substance Abuse Prevention, Substance Abuse and Mental Health Services Administration. Retrieved from http://store.samhsa.gov/shin/content/SMA10–4120/SMA10–4120.pdf

Vaillancourt, G. (2011) Music Therapists for Peace: A rebirth. *Voices: A world forum for music therapy*, Retrieved from http://testvoices.uib.no/?q=fortnightly-columns/2011-music-therapists-peace-rebirth

Valentine, E. and Evans, C. (2001) The effects of solo singing, choral singing and swimming on mood and physiological indices. *British Journal of Medical Psychology*, 74(1), 115–20.

Van Bruggen-Rufi, C. H. M. and Vink, A. C. (2011) Home is where the heart is. In A. Meadows (ed.) *Developments in Music Therapy Practice: Case study perspectives*. Gilsum, NH: Barcelona Publishers, pp. 569–82.

Van Camp, J. and De Backer, J. (2012) Autisme muzikaal! Harmonie, 'rocking', metronoom en compactheid. In G. Cluckers, C. Leroy and N. Vlieger (eds) *Het Raadsel Autisme: Psychoanalytische Psychotherapie?* Antwerp: Garant, pp. 99–115.

Van Den Hurk, J. and Smeijsters, H. (1991) Musical improvisation in the treatment of a man with obsessive compulsive personality disorder. In K. E. Bruscia (ed.) *Case Studies in Music Therapy*. Gilsum, NH: Barcelona Publishers, pp. 387–402.

Van Noorden, L. and Moelants, D. (1999) Resonance in the perception of musical pulse. *Journal of New Music Research*, 28(1), 43–66.

Verdeau-Paillès. (2005) *Le Bilan Psycho-musical et la Personnalité*, 3rd edn. Paris: Fuzeau.

Vinader, M. (2008) Music therapy: Healing, growth, and creating a culture of peace. In O. Urbain (ed.) *Music and Conflict Transformation: Harmonies and dissonances in geopolitics*. London: I. B. Tauris, pp. 147–71.

Voight, M. (2003) Orff music therapy: An overview. *Voices: A world forum for music therapy*, 3(3). Retrieved https://normt.uib.no/index.php/voices/article/view/134/110

Walworth, D. D. (2009) Effects of developmental; music groups for parents and premature of typical infants under two years on parental responsiveness and infant social development. *Journal of Music Therapy*, 46, 32–52.

Wasley, D., Williamon, A. and Taylor, A. (2011) *An Investigation into the Acute Effect of Exercise on Physiological and Psychological Responses to Musical Performance*. Paper presented at the Proceedings of the International Symposium on Performance Science.

Watzlawick, P., Helmick Beavin, J. and Jackson, D. D. (1967) *Pragmatics of Human Communication: A study of interactional patterns, pathologies, and paradoxes*. New York: W.W. Norton & Co.

Webster, J. D. and McCall, M. E. (1999) Reminiscence functions across adulthood: A replication and extension. *Journal of Adult Development*, 6, 73–85.

Weird Detroit (2011) The harmonious discord of Ira Altshuler and his musical therapy program at Eloise. Retrieved from http://weirddetroit.blogspot.com/2011/08/harmonious-discord-of-ira-altshuler-&.html

Wenger, E. (1998) *Communities of Practice: Learning, meaning, and identity*. New York: Cambridge University Press.

Wennerstrom, A. K. (2001) *The Music of Everyday Speech: Prosody and discourse analysis*. Oxford: Oxford University Press.

Wethered, A. G. (1973) *Drama and Movement in Therapy: The therapeutic use of movement, drama, and music*. London: MacDonald and Evans.

WFMT (2011) Music therapy. Retrieved from http://www.musictherapyworld.net/WFMT/About_WFMT.html

Whaley, J., Sloboda, J. and Gabrielsson, A. (2008) Peak experiences in music. In S. Hallam, I. Cross and M. Thaut (eds) *The Oxford Handbook of Music Psychology*. New York: Oxford University Press, pp. 452–61.

Wharram, B. (1969) *Elementary Rudiments of Music*. Mississauga, ON: Frederick Harris Music.

Wheeler, B. (1983) A psychotherapeutic classification of music therapy practices. *Music Therapy Perspectives*, 1(2), 8–12.

Wheeler, B. L. (1987) The use of paraverbal therapy in treating an abused child. *Arts in Psychotherapy*, 14, 69–76.

Wheeler, B. L. and Kenny, C. (2005) Principles of qualitative research. In B. L. Wheeler (ed.) *Music Therapy Research*, 2nd edn. Gilsum, NH: Barcelona Publishers, pp. 50–71.

White, M. and Epston, D. (1990) *Narrative Means to Therapeutic Ends*. New York: W.W. Norton & Co.

Wicke, P. (1991) *Rock Music: Culture, aesthetics, and sociology*. New York: Cambridge University Press.

Wigram, A. L. (1996) *The Effect of Vibroacoustic Therapy on Clinical and Non-clinical Populations*. (Doctoral dissertation). London University, London. Retrieved from http://quadrillo.tripod.com/VAT/tonyphd.html

Wigram, T. (1995) *The Art and Science of Music Therapy: A handbook*. London: Routledge.

Wigram, T. (2004) *Improvisation: Methods and techniques for music therapy clinicians, educators and students*. London: Jessica Kingsley Publishers.

Wigram, T. and Baker, F. A. (2005) Introduction: Song writing as therapy In F. A. Baker and T. Wigram (eds) *Song Writing Methods, Techniques and Clinical Applications for Music Therapy Clinicians, Educators and Students*. London: Jessica Kingsley, pp. 1–23.

Wigram, T. and De Backer, J. (eds) (1999) *Clinical Applications of Music Therapy in Psychiatry*. London: Jessica Kingsley.

Wigram, T., Pedersen, I. N. and Bonde, L. O. (2002a) *A Comprehensive Guide to Music Therapy*. London: Jessica Kingsley.

Wigram, T., Pedersen, I. N. and Bonde, L. O. (2002b) Theoretical foundations of music therapy. In T. Wigram, I. N. Pedersen and L. O. Bonde, *A Comprehensive Guide to Music Therapy: Theory, clinical practice, research, and training*. London: Jessica Kingsley, pp. 45–112.

Willis, P.R., Smith, R. and Collins, E. (eds) (2000) *Being, Seeking, Telling: Expressive approaches to qualitative adult education research*. Flaxton, Australia: Post Pressed.

Winnicott, D. W. (1953) Transitional objects and transitional phenomena. *International Journal of Psychoanalysis*, 34, 89–97.

Winnicott, D. W. (1960a) Ego distortion in terms of true and false self. *The Maturational Processes and the Facilitating Environment: Studies in the theory of emotional development*. New York: International UP, Inc, pp. 140–52.

Winnicott, D. W. (1960b) The theory of the parent–infant relationship. *International Journal of Psychoanalysis*, 41, 585–95.

Winnicott, D. W. (1965) *The Maturational Processes and the Facilitating Environment*. London: Hogarth Press and Institute of Psychoanalysis.

Winnicott, D. W. (1969) The use of an object. *International Journal of Psychoanalysis*, 50, 711–16.

Winnicott, D. W. (1971/1997) *Playing and Reality*. London: Tavistock.

Winnicott, D. W. (1974) *Gioco e Realta*. Rome: Armando.

Wolberg, L. R. (1977) *The Technique of Psychotherapy*. New York: Grune and Stratton.

Wolfgram, B. J. (1978) Music therapy for retarded adults with psychotic overlay: A day treatment approach. *Journal of Music Therapy*, 15, 199–207.

Wong, H. L., Lopez-Nahas, V. and Molassiotis, A. (2001) Effects of music therapy on anxiety in ventilator-dependent patients. *Heart and Lung*, 30(5), 376–87.

Woodcock, J. (1987) Towards group analytic music therapy. *Journal of British Music Therapy*, 1(1), 16–21.

World Health Organization (2001) *The World Health Report 2001*. (Ch. 3: Solving mental health problems). Geneva: WHO. Retrieved from http://www.who.int/whr/2001/chapter3/en/index1.html

Wosch, T. (2007) Psychology of emotion and its meaning in regulative music therapy (RT) and Guided Imagery and Music (BMGIM). In I. Frohne-Hagemann (ed.) *Receptive Music Therapy: Theory and practice*. Wiesbaden: Reichert Verlag, pp. 223–38.

Wosch, T. and Wigram, T. (eds) (2007) *Microanalysis in Music Therapy: Methods, techniques and applications for clinicians, researchers, educators, and students*. London and Philadelphia: Jessica Kingsley.

Yalom, I. D. (1980) *Existential Psychotherapy*. New York: Basic Books.

Yehuda, N. (2002) Multicultural encounters in music therapy: A qualitative research. *Nordic Journal of Music Therapy*, 2(3). Retrieved from https://normt.uib.no/index.php/voices/article/view/100/77

Yin, R. K. (2003) *Case Study Research: Design and methods*, 3rd edn. London: Sage Publications.

Young, L. (2007) Book Review: Music as therapy: A dialogical perspective [Review of *Music as Therapy: A dialogical perspective* by Rudy Garred]. *Nordic Journal of Music Therapy*, 16(1), 93.

Zadeh Mohammadi, A. (2002) *Music Therapy in Psychiatry, Medicine, and Psychology*. Tehran: Shabahang Press.

Zatorre, R. J. and Belin, P. (2001) Spectral and temporal processing in human auditory cortex. *Cerebral Cortex*, 11(10), 946–53.

Zbikowski, L. M. (2011) *Music, Language, and What Falls in Between*. Chicago, IL: University of Chicago Department of Music.

Zeanah, C. H. and Zeanah, P. D. (2009) The scope of infant mental health. In C.H. Zeanah (ed.) *Handbook of Infant Mental Health*. New York: Guilford Press, pp. 5–21.

Zinberg, N. (1977) The study of consciousness states: Problems and progress. In N. Zinberg (ed.) *Alternate States of Consciousness*. New York: Free Press.

Zwerling, I. (1989) The creative arts therapies as 'real therapies'. *American Journal of Dance Therapy*, 11(1), 19–26.